The
Charles Press

Handbook of Current Medical Abbreviations

Fifth Edition

The Charles Press Handbook of Current Medical Abbreviations

Fifth Edition

The Charles Press, Publishers
Philadelphia

The Charles Press, Publishers
Post Office Box 15715
Philadelphia, PA 19103
(215) 496-9616 - Telephone
(215) 496-9637 - Fax
mailbox@charlespresspub.com

Library of Congress Cataloging-in-Publication Data

The Charles Press handbook of current medical abbreviations — 5th ed.
p. cm.
ISBN 0-914783-81-5 (pbk. alk. paper)
1. Medicine — Abbreviations. I. Charles Press Publishers.
[DNLM: 1. Medicine — Abbreviations. W 13 C476 1997]
R123.C442 1997
610'.1'48 — dc21
DNLM/DLC
for Library of Congress
97-12402

Printed in Canada

Second Printing

A

A	absolute temperature absorbance (radiology) adult alive amalgam (dentistry) ambulatory area artery assessment average axial
Ⓐ	axillary
a	accommodation (eye examination) acid after agar ampere anode anterior water (Latin: *aqua*)
$\mathbf{A_1}$, $\mathbf{A_2}$	aortic heart sounds (first, second)
$\bar{\mathbf{a}}$	before (Latin: *ante*) of each
AA	acetic acid achievement age (pediatrics) active assistance (orthopedics) acute asthma alcohol abuse Alcoholics Anonymous amino acid antiarrhythmic agent anticipatory avoidance aortic aneurysm

AA *(cont)*	aplastic anemia arachidonic acid arm-ankle (pulse ratio) ascending aorta atomic absorption Australia antigen authorized absence automobile accident
A-a	alveolar-arterial (gradient)
aa or $\bar{a}\bar{a}$	of each (medication orders)
AAA	abdominal aortic aneurysm acquired aplastic anemia acute anxiety attack amalgam amino acid analysis androgenic anabolic agent
AAAAA	aphasia, agnosia, apraxia, agraphia, alexia
AAC	antibiotic-associated colitis antigen-antibody crossed electrophoresis
AACE	antimicrobial agents and chemotherapy
AAD	alpha antitrypsin deficiency antibiotic-associated diarrhea
A-aDO_2	alveolar-arterial oxygen difference
AADR	age-adjusted death rate
AAE	active assistive exercise acute allergic encephalitis
AAF	ascorbic acid factor
AAGS	adult adrenogenital syndrome

AAH	aortic arch hypoplasia
AAI	acute adrenal insufficiency arm-ankle indices
AAIA	acquired artery immune augmentation
AAL	anterior axillary line
AAMD	age-associated memory disorder
AAME	acetyl argenine methyl ester
AAMS	acute aseptic meningitis syndrome
AAN	amino acid nitrogen
AAO	amino acid oxidase
$(A\text{-}a)O_2$	alveolar-arterial oxygen gradient
AAOx3	awake and oriented to time, place and person
AAP	acute apical periodontitis air at atmospheric pressure
AAPCC	adjusted average per capita cost
$(A\text{-}a)P_{CO2}$	alveolar-arterial pulmonary carbon dioxide gradient
AAPMC	antibiotic-associated pseudomembranous colitis
AAR	antigen-antiglobulin reaction Australia antigen radioimmunoassay
AARF	acute alveolar respiratory failure

AAS	acute abdominal series anabolic-androgenic steroid anthrax antiserum aortic arch syndrome atomic absorption spectrophotometry
AASH	adrenal androgen stimulating hormone
AAT	acute abdominal tympany alpha-1 antitrypsin auditory apperception test
AAU	acute anterior uveitis
AAV	adeno-associated virus
AB	Ace Bandage aid to the blind alcian blue apex beat asthmatic bronchitis axiobuccal (dentistry)
A/B	acid-base ratio apnea/bradycardia (moderate stimulation)
A & B	apnea and bradycardia
A>B	air greater than bone conduction
Ab	antibody abortion
ABA	allergic bronchopulmonary aspergillosis antibacterial activity
ABC	abbreviated blood count airway, breathing, circulation apnea, bradycardia, cyanosis applesauce, bananas, cereal (diet)

ABCX	adriamycin, bleomycin, cisplatin and radiation therapy
ABD	aged, blind, disabled
abd	abdomen abduction
ABE	acute bacterial endocarditis
ABEP	auditory brainstem evoked potential
ABF	aortobifemoral (bypass)
ABG	arterial blood gas
AbH	abdominal hysterectomy
ABI	ankle-brachial index atherosclerotic brain infarction
ABL	abetalipoproteinemia antigen-binding lymphocytes axiobuccolingual (dentistry)
ABLB	alternate binaural loudness balance (test)
ABMT	autologous bone marrow transplantation
Abn	abnormal
ABO	absent bed occupant
ABP	arterial blood pressure
ABPA	acute bronchopulmonary asthma
ABPM	ambulatory blood pressure monitoring
ABR	abrasion

ABR *(cont)*	absolute bed rest auditory brainstem response
ABS	abdominal surgery acute brain syndrome admitting blood sugar
abs	absent absolute
ABT	autologous bone marrow transplantation
ABVD	adriamycin, bleomycin, vinblastine, dacarbazine
ABW	actual body weight
abx	antibiotics
aby	antibody
AC	abdominal circumference adenocarcinoma adrenal cortex air conduction (hearing test) alcoholic coma alternating current anterior chamber (eye examination) anterior colporrhaphy (gynecology) anticoagulant aortic closure assist control
A/C	albumin-coagulin ratio ambulatory care anchored catheter
ac	acid acute before meals (Latin: *ante cibum*)

ACA	achylic chloroanemia adenocarcinoma anterior cerebral artery
ACB	alveolar capillary block
ACBE	air-contrast barium enema
ACBGS	aortocoronary bypass graft surgery
ACBS	aortocoronary bypass surgery
ACC	adenoid cystic carcinoma ambulatory care center anodal closure contraction
acc	accident according
accom	accommodation (eye examination)
ACD	absolute cardiac dullness adult celiac disease anterior chest diameter anticonvulsant drug
ACDF	adult child of dysfunctional family anterior cervical discectomy and fusion
ACE	alcoholic cardiomegaly-emphysema angiotensin-converting enzyme
ACF	accessory clinical findings acid-fast culture acute care facility
ACG	angiocardiogram angle closure glaucoma apexcardiogram

ACH	adrenal cortical hormone arm, chest, height
ACh	acetylcholine
ACI	acute coronary insufficiency adenylate cyclase inhibitor aftercare instructions
ACIDS	acquired cellular immunodeficient syndrome
ACJ	acromioclavicular joint
ACM	Arnold-Chiari malformation
ACOA	adult child of alcoholic
ACP	acyl-carrier protein adnodal closing picture aspirin, caffeine, phenacetin
ac phos	acid phosphatase
ACPP	adrenocorticopolypeptide
ACPPD	average cost per patient day
ACR	adjusted community rating anticonstipation regimen
ACS	ambulatory care services anodal closing sound antireticular cytotoxic serum
acs	amniocentesis
ACSV	aortocoronary saphenous vein (graft)
ACT	activated clotting time

ACT *(cont)*	anticoagulant therapy
ACTA	automatic computerized transverse axial (scans)
ACTD	actinomycin D
ACTG	AIDS Clinical Trials Group
ACTH	adrenocorticotropic hormone
ACTN	adrenocorticotrophin
ACTP	adrenocorticotropic polypeptide
ACU	acute care unit ambulatory care unit
ACV	acyclovir
ACVD	acute cardiovascular disease autoimmune collagen vascular disease
AD	admitting diagnosis advance directive after discharge alcohol dehydrogenase alternating days Alzheimer's disease analgesic dose right ear (Latin: *auris dextra*)
Ad	adrenal
ad	adnexa
ADA diet	American Diabetes Association diet
ADB	accidental death benefit (insurance)

ADC	adult day care albumin, dextrose, catalase anodal duration contraction
AdC	adenylate cyclase adrenal cortex
ADD	attention deficit disorder average daily dose
Add	adduction
ADDU	alcohol and drug dependency unit
ADE	acute disseminated encephalitis
ADEM	acute disseminated encephalomyelitis
ADG	atrial diastolic gallop
ADH	alcohol dehydrogenase antidiuretic hormone
ADHD	attention-deficit hyperactivity disorder
ADI	acceptable daily intake
adj	adjustment
ADL	activities of daily living adolescent medicine
ad lib	as desired (Latin: *ad libitum*)
ADM	adriamycin
adm	admission
adol	adolescent

ADP	adenosine diphosphate area diastolic pressure
ADR	absence of deep reflexes adverse drug reaction
ADRD	Alzheimer's disease and related disorders
ADS	anonymous donor sperm antibody deficient syndrome antidiuretic substance
ADSU	ambulatory diagnostic surgery unit
ADT	accepted dental therapeutics adenosine triphosphate alternate day treatment
ADTP	alcohol dependency treatment program
A-DV	arterial-deep venous (difference)
AdV	adenovirus
AE	above elbow air entry (pulmonary medicine)
AEA	above-elbow amputation allergic extrinsic alveolitis
AED	antiepileptic drug automatic external defibrillator
AEG	air encephalogram
AEL	acute erythroleukemia
AEP	admission evaluation protocol
AEq	age equivalent (pediatrics)

AER	albumin excretion rate auditory evoked response
AES	Alzheimer's euphoria state antieosinophilic serum
AET	absorption equivalent thickness
AF	acid-fast amniotic fluid aortic flow Asian female atrial fibrillation
Af	atrial flutter
AFA	alcohol-formalin-acetic acid
AFB	acid-fast bacillus
AFBG	aortofemoral bypass graft
AFD	assessment of fat distribution
AFH	adenofibromatous hyperplasia
A fib	atrial fibrillation
AFO	ankle-foot orthosis (splint)
AFP	alpha-fetoprotein atrial filling pressure
AFRD	acute febrile respiratory disease
AFS	acid-fast smear Alzheimer's fugue state
AFV	amniotic fluid volume

AFX	air-fluid exchange atypical fibroxanthoma
AG	anion gap antiglobulin
A/G	albumin-globulin ratio
Ag	antigen
AGA	acute gonococcal arthritis appropriate for gestational age
AGC	absolute granulocyte count
AGD	agar gel diffusion
AGE	acute gastroenteritis angle of greatest extension
AGF	angle of greatest flexion
AGG	agammaglobulinemia
aggl	agglutination
AGH	amenorrhea-galactorrhea hypothyroidism
agit	shake (Latin: *agita*)
AGL	acute granulocytic leukemia
AGN	acute glomerulonephritis agnosia
$AgNO_3$ sol	silver nitrate solution
AGPT	agar gel precipitation test
AGS	adrenogenital syndrome

AGT	antiglobulin test
AGTT	abnormal glucose tolerance test
AH	accidental hypothermia acute hepatitis aqueous humor (eye) arterial hypertension
Ah	hypermetropic astigmatism
AHA	abortive hereditary ataxia acquired hemolytic anemia autoimmune hemolytic anemia
AHC	acute hemorrhagic cystitis
AHD	antihypertensive drug arteriosclerotic heart disease autoimmune hemolytic disease
AHE	acute hemorrhagic encephalomyelitis
AHF	acute heart failure antihemophilic factor
AHG	antihemophilic globulin
AHIP	assisted health insurance plan
AHM	ambulatory Holter monitoring apical holosystolic murmur (cardiology)
AHN	assistant head nurse
AHNS	arteriolar hyperplastic nephrosclerosis
AHP	Accountable Health Plan
AI	accidental injury

AI *(cont)*	allergy and immunology anxiety index aortic insufficiency apnea index artificial insemination atrial insufficiency autoimmune
A & I	allergy and immunology
AICD	automatic implantable cardioverter/defibrillator
AID	acute infectious disease anti-inflammatory drug artificial insemination donor autoimmune disease
AIDS	acquired immune deficiency syndrome
AIE	acute infective endocarditis
AIF	anti-invasion factor
AIG	anti-immunoglobulin
AIH	artificial insemination by husband
AIL	angioimmunoblastic lymphadenopathy
AILC	adult independent living center
AIMS	abnormal involuntary movement scale
AIN	acute intersitial nephritis
AIP	acute idiopathic pericarditis acute intermittent porphyria average intravascular pressure

AIR	accelerated idioventricular rhythm
AIS	anti-insulin serum
AIU	absolute iodine uptake
AJ	ankle jerk
AKA	apple juice only
AK	above knee (amputation) actinic keratosis
AKA	alcoholic ketoacidosis
AL	adaptation level arterial line axiolingual
ALAD	abnormal left axis deviation (cardiology)
alb	albumin
ALC	absolute lymphocyte count approximate lethal concentration
ALD	adrenoleukodystrophy alcohol liver disease
ALE	allowable limits of error
ALFT	abnormal liver function tests
ALG	antilymphocytic globulin
ALHE	agniolymphoid hyperplasia with eosinophilia
A-line	arterial line

alk	alkaline
alk phos	alkaline phosphatase
ALL	acute lymphocytic leukemia
ALM	adhesive leptomeningitis alveolar lining material
ALN	anterior lymph node
ALO	acute laryngeal obstruction
ALOH	average length of hospitalization
ALQTS	acquired long QT syndrome (ECG report)
ALRI	acute lower respiratory infection
ALS	acute lateral sclerosis advanced life support amyotrophic lateral sclerosis
ALT	alanine aminotransferase (enzyme)
ALTE	apparent life-threatening event
alt	alternate
alv	alveolar
AM	aerospace medicine anovular menstruation arterial mean Asian male Austin-Moore (prosthesis) before noon (Latin: *ante meridianus*)
AMA	against medical advice antimitochondrial antibody

AMAP	as much as possible
AMB	amphotericin B
amb	ambulate
AMBL	acute myeloblastic leukemia
AMG	aminoglycoside
AMH	automated medical history
AMHT	automated multiphasic health testing
AMI	acute myocardial infarction
AML	acute myelogenous leukemia automated Medicare log
AMLR	autologous mixed lymphocyte reaction
amm	ammonia
AMN	angiomyoneuroma
amor	amorphous
AMP	adenosine monophosphate ampicillin average mean pressure
amp	ampere ampule (medical order) amputation
amph	amphetamine
AMR	alternating motor rate
AMRS	automated medical record system

AMS	acute mountain sickness admission multiphasic screening aggravated in military service altered mental status automated multiphasic screening
amt	amount
AMV	assisted mechanical ventilation
AMVI	acute mesenteric vascular insufficiency
AMVL	anterior mitral valve leaflet
AMX	amoxicillin
AN	anesthesia aneurysm anorexia nervosa aseptic necrosis
ANA	antinuclear antibody
ANAD	anorexia nervosa and associated disorders
ANB	atrioventricular nodal block
ANCA	antineutrophil cytoplasmic antibody
AnCC	anodal closure contraction
AND	anorexia, nausea, diarrhea anterior nasal discharge
ANDA	Abbreviated New Drug Application
ANF	antinuclear factor
ang	angiogram

anh	anhydrous
aniso	anisocytosis (of red blood cells)
ANLL	acute nonlymphocytic leukemia
ANS	acute nephritic syndrome anterior nasal spine arteriolonephrosclerosis autonomic nervous system
ANT	acoustic noise test
ant	anterior
ant ax	anterior axillary line
ANUG	acute necrotizing ulcerative gingivitis
ANV	anorexia, nausea, vomiting
AO	acid output anodal opening anterior oblique
A&O	alert and oriented
AOAP	as often as possible
AOB	alcohol on breath assignment of benefits
AOC	abridged ocular chart
AOD	arterial occlusive disease arterial oxygen desaturation auriculoosteodysplasia azotemic osteodystrophy
AODM	adult onset diabetes mellitus

AOL	acroosteolysis (distal phalangeal resorption)
AOM	acute otitis media
AoP	left ventricle to aorta pressure gradient
AOS	Agent Orange syndrome anodal opening sound
AP	action potential (cardiology) acute phase alkaline phosphatase alum-precipitated angina pectoris antepartum anterior pituitary anteroposterior aortic pressure apical pulse appendectomy artificial pneumothorax attending physician
A/P	ascites-plasma (ratio)
A & P	anatomy and physiology anterior and posterior auscultation and percussion
A2>P2	aortic second sound is greater than pulmonic second sound
APA	acute pain attack aldosterone-producing adenoma
APACHE	acute physiology and chronic health evaluation
APAS	annular phased array system (cardiology)

APB	atrial premature beat
APC	adenomatous polyposis coli antigen presenting cell atrial premature contraction
APC tabs	aspirin, phenacetin and caffeine tablets
APD	abdominal postoperative dehiscence action potential duration ambulatory peritoneal dialysis anteroposterior diameter arteriopathic dementia atrial premature depolarization
APE	acute psychotic episode acute pulmonary edema
APF	aortopulmonary fistula
APG	ambulatory patient group
APH	antepartum hemorrhage (obstetrics) anterior pituitary hormone
APKD	adult polycystic kidney disease
APL	accelerated painless labor
A-P & L	anterior-posterior and lateral (x-ray/chest)
APM	anterior papillary muscle anteroposterior movement
APN	acute pyelonephritis arsenic polyneuropathy
APO	apomorphine
APP	alum-precipitated protein

appl	appliance application applied
appt	appointment
APPX	appendix
APR	abdominoperineal resection acute pain reaction average payment rate
A-PR	anterior-posterior repair
APSAC	anisoylated plasminogen streptokinase activator complex
APSD	aorticopulmonary septal defect
APT	alum-precipitated toxoid arsenic pseudotabes auricular paroxysmal tachycardia
APTT	activated partial thromboplastin time
APUD	amine precursor uptake and decarboxylation
APVD	anomalous pulmonary venous drainage
APVM	acute perivascular myelinoclasis
AQ	achievement quotient (psychiatry)
aq	aqueous
aq dist	distilled water (Latin: *aqua distillata*)
AR	active resistance (exercise) adverse reaction

AR *(cont)*	allergic rhinitis aortic regurgitation apical rate artificial respiration
A/R	apical/radial (pulse)
A & R	advised and released
ARB	any reliable brand (prescriptions)
ARBD	alcohol-related birth defect
ARC	AIDS-related complex alcohol rehabilitation center
ARD	acute respiratory disease anorectal dressing arthritis and rheumatic diseases
ARDS	adult respiratory distress syndrome
ARF	acute renal failure acute respiratory failure acute rheumatic fever
ARI	acute respiratory infection
ARLD	alcohol-related liver disease
ARM	allergy relief medicine arteriovenous malformation
ARMD	age-related macular degeneration
AROA	autosomal recessive ocular albinism
AROM	active range of motion artificial rupture of the membranes

ARP	at-risk period
arr	arrive
ARS	antirabies serum
ART	acoustic reflex test automated reagin test
art	artifact (laboratory/chemistry)
ARV	AIDS-related virus anterior right ventricular (wall)
AS	active sleep antiserum aortic stenosis aqueous solution arteriosclerosis left ear (Latin: *auris sinistra*)
As	astigmatism
ASA	acetylsalicylic acid (aspirin) Adams-Stokes attack antibody to surface antigen
ASAP	as soon as possible
ASAT	aspartate aminotransferase
ASB	anesthesia standby
ASC	altered state of consciousness Ancell-Spiegler cylindroma apical systolic click (cardiology)
ASCVD	arteriosclerotic cardiovascular disease

ASD	Adams-Stokes disease atrial septal defect
ASDH	acute subdural hematoma
ASE	axilla, shoulder, elbow (bandage)
ASH	asymmetrical septal hypertrophy
AsH	hypermetropic astigmatism
ASHD	arteriosclerotic heart disease
ASHN	acute sclerosing hyaline necrosis
ASIA	angiosclerotic intermittent akinesia
ASID	angiosclerotic intermittent dyskinesia
ASK	antistreptokinase
ASL	American Sign Language antistreptolysin
ASM	myopic astigmatism
ASN	acquired splenic neutropenia
ASO	administrative services on (contract) antistreptolysin-O (titer) atherosclerosis obliterans
ASP	alkaline serum phosphatase
ASPD	antisocial personality disorder
ASPM	angiosclerotic paroxysmal myasthenia
ASR	age/sex rates aldosterone secretion rate

ASS	acute serum sickness anterior superior spine assessment
assoc	associated
AST	aspartate aminotransferase
Ast	astigmatism
as tol	as tolerated
ASU	ambulatory surgical unit
ASV	antisnake venom
ASVD	arterial-superficial venous difference arteriosclerotic vascular disease
Asx	asymptomatic
AT	activity therapist adjunctive therapy adjuvant therapy air temperature antithrombin applantation tonometry atrial tachycardia
ATA	antithyroglobulin antibody
ATB	atrial tachycardia with block
ATC	around the clock
ATD	Alzheimer's type dementia
ATF	absence of typical findings
ATG	antithymocyte globulin

ATL	Achilles tendon lengthening atypical lymphocytes
ATN	acute tubular necrosis
ATP	addiction treatment program adenosine triphosphate ambient temperature and pressure anatomic pathology
ATR	Achilles tendon reflex
atr	atrophy
ATS	antitetanic serum apathetic thyrotoxic storm atherosclerosis
$ATSO_4$	atropine sulfate
ATT	arginine tolerance test
AU	both ears (Latin: *aures unites*)
^{198}Au	radioactive gold (nuclear medicine)
AUD	auditory
Aud comp	auditory compensation
AUL	acute undifferentiated leukemia
AUTI	asymptomatic urinary tract infection
aux	auxiliary
AV	adriamycin and vincristine (chemotherapy) aortic valve arbovirus arteriovenous

AV *(cont)*	assisted ventilation atrioventricular
AVA	aortic valve atresia
AVB	abnormal vaginal bleeding atrioventricular block
AVC	aortic valve closure
AVD	aortic valve disease
$AVDO_2$	arteriovenous oxygen difference
aVF	augmented V lead, left leg (ECG)
AVGs	ambulatory visit groups
AVH	acute viral hepatitis
aVL	augmented V lead, left arm (ECG)
AVM	adriamycin, vinblastine, methotrexate arteriovenous malformation
AVN	atrioventricular node
AVNB	atrioventricular nodal block
AVO_2	arteriovenous oxygen difference
AVOC	avocation
AVP	adriamycin, vinblastine, procarbazine antiviral protein
AVR	aortic valve replacement
aVR	augmented V lead, right arm (ECG)

AVRT	atrioventricular reentrant tachycardia
AVS	arteriovenous shunt
AVSS	afebrile, vital signs stable
AVT	atypical ventricular tachycardia
AW	anterior wall
A/W	able to walk
A & W	alive and well
aw	airways
A waves	atrial contraction waves
AWDW	assault with a deadly weapon
AWMI	anterior wall myocardial infarction
AWP	airway pressure average wholesale price
AWS	alcohol withdrawal syndrome
Ax	axillary
AXR	abdominal x-ray
AXT	alternating extropia
ax	axis
AZT	azidothymidine (AIDS treatment drug)

B

B	bacillus bicuspid (dentistry) black both brother Brucella (on bacteriology reports) buccal (surface) blood
b	born
BA	basilar artery biliary atony bile acid blood agar (culture medium) blood alcohol bone age (radiology) brachial artery bronchial asthma
Ba	barium
B/A	backache
BAB	blood agar base
Bab	Babinski sign (neurology)
BAC	blood alcohol concentration
BACOP	bleomycin, adriamycin, cyclophosphamide, oncovin, prednisone (chemotherapy)
bact	bacteria
BaE	barium enema (x-ray/colon)
BAEP	brainstem auditory evoked potential

BAER	brainstem auditory evoked response
BAF	breast adenofibroma
BAL	blood alcohol level British anti-lewisite (medication order) bronchial alveolar lavage (pulmonary procedure)
BALT	bronchus-associated lymphoid tissue
BAm	mean brachial artery (pressure)
bands	banded neutrophilis
BAO	basal acid output
BAP	body adiposity percentage brachial artery pressure
barb	barbiturate
BASH	body acceleration synchronous with heartbeat
baso	basophils
Ba swal	barium swallow (x-ray/esophagus)
BAT	best available technology brown adipose tissue
BAV	balloon aortic valvuloplasty
BB	bath blanket bed bath beta-blocker blood bank both bones (regarding fractures) breakthrough bleeding

BB *(cont)*	brush border buffer base
BBA	born before arrival
BBB	baseball bat beating blood-brain barrier bundle branch block (ECG)
BBBB	bilateral bundle branch block (ECG)
BBM	banked breast milk
BBR	bibasilar rales (cardiology)
BBS	bilateral breath sounds
BBT	basal body temperature
BBx	breast biopsy
BC	basal cell battered child birth control blood culture Blue Cross board-certified bone conduction (hearing test) Bowman's capsule (nephrology)
B & C	bed and chair (rest) biopsy and curettage board and care
BCA	balloon catheter angioplasty body composition analysis brachiocephalic artery
BCAA	branched chain amino acid

BCAT	breast changes and tenderness
BCBE	board certified/board eligible
BC/BS	Blue Cross/Blue Shield
BCC	basal cell carcinoma birth control clinic
BCD	basal cell dyplasia
BCDDP	Breast Cancer Detection Demonstration Program
BCE	barium contrast enema basal cell epithelioma
BCF	basophil chemotactic factor
BCG	bacille Calmette-Guérin (vaccine)
BCH	basal cell hyperplasia
BCLS	basic cardiac life support
BCM	birth control medication
BCMD	benign congenital muscular dystrophy
BCN	basal cell nevus (dermatology) bilateral cortical necrosis
BCP	birth control pills
BCS	battered child syndrome
BCSI	breast cancer screening indicator
BCSP	breast cystosarcoma phylloides

BCT	breast conserving treatment (oncology)
BCU	burn care unit
BD	behavioral disorder bile duct birth defect blood donor bottle drainage brain dead
BDC	burn dressing change
BDD	balanced-deficit diet bed-disability day body dysmorphic disorder
BDI	Beck Depression Inventory (psychiatry)
BDM	beer drinkers' myocardiopathy
bDNA	branched DNA (test/HIV)
BE	bacterial endocarditis barium enema (x-ray/colon) below elbow (operation/amputation) board-eligible brain edema
BEA	bronchitis, emphysema, asthma
BEAM	brain electrical activity mapping
BEC	bacterial endocarditis
BED	binge eating disorder
BEE	basal energy expenditure

BEI	butanol extractable iodine (laboratory/thyroid chemistry)
BEP	brainstem evoked potential
BET	benign epithelial tumor
bev	billion electron volts (radiation therapy)
BEW	blood and electrolyte work-up
BF	black female blood flow body fat bone fragment breast-feed
B/F	bound-free (antigen ratio)
BFB	bifascicular block (electrocardiogram)
BFBM	birefringent foreign body material (forensic pathology)
BFC	benign febrile convulsion
BFD	body fat distribution
BFM	black female, married
BFP	biological false positive (test)
BFR	blood flow rate bone formation rate
BFRS	buffered Ringer's solution (intravenous solution)
BFT	bentonite flocculation test Brooke-Fordyce trichoepithelioma

BG	basal ganglion Bender Gestalt (psychiatric test) blood glucose (laboratory/chemistry) bone graft (operation/orthopedics)
BGC	blood glucose concentration
BGG	bovine gammaglobulin
BHC	Braxton-Hicks contraction (obstetrics)
BHI	bone healing index
BHL	biologic half-life
BHR	basal heart rate
BHS	beta-hemolytic streptococcus
BH/VH	body hematocrit-venous hematocrit ratio
BI	bladder insufficiency bodily injury (emergency medicine) bone injury brain injury burn index
BIA	bicarbonate ingestion alkalosis
BIB	brought in by (hospital arrival)
bib	drink (Latin: *bibe*) (medication order)
BID	body image disturbance brought in dead
bid	twice a day (Latin: *bis in die*)
BIH	benign intracranial hypertension

BIL	basal insulin level
bilat	bilateral
bili	bilirubin (laboratory/chemistry)
bili-C	conjugated bilirubin
bili-D/I	direct and indirect bilirubin
bili-T	total bilirubin
BIN	benign intradermal nevus
BIP	bacterial intravenous protein
BIR	basic incidence rate
BISp	between ischial spines (pelvic measurement)
bisp diam	bispinous diameter (pelvic measurement)
BJ	biceps jerk bone and joint
BJM	bones, joints, muscles
BJP	Bence Jones protein (laboratory/urine)
BKA	below knee amputation
bkfst	breakfast
BKTT	below knee to toe (cast)
BKWC	below knee walking cast
BL	baseline blood loss

BL *(cont)*	borderline bronchial lavage Burkitt's lymphoma
Bl	black
bl	bleeding blood blue
BLAD	borderline left axis deviation (cardiology)
BLB	blood bank Boothby-Lovelace-Bulbulian (mask)
blc	blood culture (laboratory/bacteriology)
BLD	bilateral deafness
BLE	both lower extremities
bleo	bleomycin
BLESS	bath, laxative, enema, shampoo, shower
BLFG	bilateral firm (hand) grips
BLJ	black liver jaundice
BLL	brows, lids, lashes
BLLS	bilateral leg strength
BLN	bronchial lymph nodes
BLP	bilateral papilledema
BLR	base line record (dentistry)
BLS	basic life support

BLT	bilateral tubal (ligation) blood (clot) lysis time
BlT	blood type
blx	bleeding time
BM	basal metabolism basement membrane black male body mass bone marrow bowel movement breast milk buccal mass (dentistry)
BMAB	bone marrow aspirate and biopsy
BMC	bone marrow cells
BMD	bone marrow depression
BMET	biomedical electronics technician
BMG	benign monoclonal gammopathy
BMH	bone marrow hypoplasia
BMI	body mass index
BMJ	bones, muscles, joints breast milk jaundice
BMK	birthmark
BMN	bone marrow necrosis
BMR	basal metabolic rate

BMT	behavioral marital therapy bone marrow transplant
BMV	billowing mitral valve (cardiology)
BMZ	basement membrane zone
BN	bladder neck brachial neuritis
BNC	bladder neck contracture (urology)
BNDD	Bureau of Narcotics and Dangerous Drugs (precedes physician's narcotic number)
bne	but not exceeding (dose)
BNO	bladder neck obstruction (urology)
BO	body odor bowel obstruction
B/O	because of bowels open
BOA	behavior observation audiometry born on arrival
BOC	blood oxygen capacity
BOD	biochemical oxygen demand
BOE	bilateral otitis externa
BOL	blood oxygen level
bol	bolus (medication orders/prescriptions)
BOM	bilateral otitis media

BOP	bleomycin, oncovin, prednisone (chemotherapy)
BOR	bowels open regularly
BO_2S	blood oxygen saturation
BOT	base of tongue benign ovarian tumor
BOW	bag of waters (obstetrics)
BP	back pressure bathroom privileges bedpan Bell's palsy birthplace blood pressure body part bronchopleural bypass (operation/cardiovascular)
BPAD	bipolar affective disorder
BPD	biparietal diameter (obstetrics) blood pressure decreased borderline personality disorder bronchopulmonary dysplasia
BPF	bronchopleural fistula
BPG	blood pressure gauge
BPH	benign prostatic hypertrophy
BPI	bipolar illness (psychiatry) blood pressure increased
BPLND	bilateral pelvic lymph node dissection

BPM	beats per minute
BPOB	bile pigment (hourly) output of bilirubin (diagnostic procedure)
BPOL	bilateral parietooccipital lesion
BPP	brachial plexus paralysis
BPPV	benign paroxysmal positional vertigo
BPR	blood pressure reading
BPS	beats per second
BPV	benign paroxysmal vertigo
BR	bathroom bedrest
Br	breech bridge (dentistry) bromide brown
BRAT	bananas, rice, applesauce, toast (diet)
BRB	blood retinal barrier bright red blood
BRM	biological response modifier
BrM	breast milk
BRO	bronchoscopy
BRP	bathroom privileges
BrT	breast tumor

BRVO	branch retinal vein occlusion
BS	Babinski sign bedside before sleep blood sugar Blue Shield
B/S	breath sounds
b/s	bowel sounds
B & S	Bartholin and Skene glands
BSA	body surface area both sexes affected
BSB	body surface burned
BSC	bedside commode
BSD	bedside drainage
BSE	breast self-examination
BSER	brainstem evoked response
BSF	basal skull fracture
BSI	bound serum iron
BSL	blood sugar level brainstem lesion
BSN	bowel sounds normal
BSO	bilateral salpingo-oophorectomy (operation/gynecology)
BSOM	bilateral serous otitis media

BSp	bronchospasm
BSR	basal skin resistance blood sedimentation rate
BSS	black silk sutures buffered saline solution
BS/ST	brain scan/spinal tap
BST	breast stimulation test brief stimulus therapy
BSU	British standard unit
BT	bedtime bladder tumor body temperature body type brain tumor
BTB	breakthrough bleeding bromthymol blue (laboratory)
BTFS	breast tumor frozen section
BTL	bilateral tubal ligation (operation/gynecology)
BTPD	body temperature and ambient pressure, dry (in pulmonary function test reports)
BTPS	body temperature and ambient pressure, saturated with water vapor (in pulmonary function test reports)
BTR	bladder tumor recheck (urology)
BTU	British thermal unit

BU	below umbilicus blood urea burn unit
BUA	blood uric acid
BUE	both upper extremities
BUI	brain uptake index
BUN	blood urea nitrogen
BUO	bleeding of undetermined origin
BV	blood volume bronchovesicular (breath sounds)
B/V	binging and vomiting
bv	blood vessel
BVAD	biventricular assistive device
BVDT	brief vesticular disorientation test (neurology)
BVE	biventricular enlargement
BVH	biventricular hypertrophy (heart)
BVL	bilateral vas ligation (operation/genitourinary)
BVRT	Benton Visual Retention Test
BVTA	biventricular transposed aorta
BW	below waist birth weight body water body weight

BWCS	bagged white cell study
BWS	battered woman syndrome
BWX	bitewing x-ray (dentistry)
Bx	biopsy

C

C	ascorbic acid calorie carbohydrate carrier Catholic Caucasian Celsius (temperature) certified cesarean (section) cervical chest chloramphenicol cholesterol clearance closure cocaine coefficient concentration contraction correct cylinder (eye examination) hundred (Latin: *centum*)
©	confidential
c	approximately (Latin: *circa*) canine (dentistry) capacity capillary cubic
C'	complement
C_1 to C_7	cervical vertebrae 1 through 7
C-I to C-V	controlled substances (Schedules I through V)

c̄	with (Latin: *cum*)
CA	cancer carbonic anhydrase carcinoma (cancer) cardiac arrest cardiac arrhythmia carotid artery cholic acid chronological age citric acid Cocaine Anonymous cold agglutinin common antigen congenital anomaly corneal abrasion coronary angioplasty coronary arrest coronary artery cortisone acetate
C/A	canceled appointment
Ca	calcium carcinoma carpal amputation cathode
[Ca^{++}]	intracellular free calcium concentration
ca	about (Latin: *circa*)
c/a	Clinitest/Acetest
CAA	computer-assisted assessment crystalline amino acids
CaAd	adenocarcinoma
CAB	coronary artery bypass

CABG	coronary artery bypass graft
CABP	calcium-binding protein
CAC	cardiac arrest code circulating anticoagulant comprehensive ambulatory care
CACC	cathodal closure contraction
CACG	cineangiocardiogram
CACI	computer-assisted continous infusion
CaCx	cancer of the cervix
CAD	cadaver computer-assisted diagnosis coronary artery disease
CADL	Communicative Abilities in Daily Living
CAF	continuous atrial fibrillation contract administration fees coronary arteriovenous fistula cyclophosphamide, adriamycin, fluorouracil (chemotherapy)
Caf	caffeine
CAG	chronic atrophic gastritis
CAH	chronic active hepatitis congenital adrenal hyperplasia
CAHC	chronic active hepatitis with cirrhosis
CAHJ	cup arthroplasty of the hip joint
CAHS	central alveolar hypoventilation syndrome

CAI	calcium intake computer-assisted instruction confused artificial insemination
CaI	carotid artery insufficiency
Cal	caliber
cal	calorie
$\mathbf{C_{alb}}$	albumin clearance
calc	calculate
cal ct	calorie count
CALD	chronic active liver disease
CALH	chronic active lupoid hepatitis
CALLA	common acute lymphocytic leukemia antigen
CAM	Caucasian adult male computer-assisted myelography
$\mathbf{C_{am}}$	amylase clearance
CAMAC	computer-assisted measurement and control
CAMP	Christie-Atkins-Munch-Peterson (test) computer-assisted menu planning
cAMP	cyclic adenosine monophosphate
CAMS	computerized arrythmia monitoring system
CAMU	cardiac arrhythmia monitoring unit

CAN	child abuse and neglect cord (umbilical) around neck
CANS	central auditory nervous system
CAO	carotid artery occlusion chronic airway obstruction
CAP	capitation (risk-sharing reimbursement) catabolite activator protein cell attachment protein cholesteric analysis profile chronic alcoholic pancreatitis chronic apical periodontitis compound action potential
CaP	prostate cancer
cap	capillary
CAPA	caffeine, alcohol, pepper, aspirin (diet free of)
CAPD	continuous ambulatory peritoneal dialysis
CAPERS	Computer-assisted Psychiatric Evaluation and Review System
caps	capsules
CAPYA	child and adolescent psychoanalysis
CAR	cardiac ambulation routine chronic articular rheumatism
CARA	congenital aregenerative anemia
CART	computer-assisted real-time transcription
CAS	carotid artery stenosis (stroke)

CAS *(cont)*	congenital alcohol syndrome
CASF	coronary arteriosystemic fistula
CASP	calcium urine spot (test)
CaSq	squamous cell carcinoma
CAST	color allergy screening test
CAT	computerized axial tomography computerized transcription
cath	cathartic catheter
caut	cauterize
CAV	congenital absence of vagina congenital adrenal virilism croup-associated virus
CAVB	complete atrioventricular block
CAVH	continuous arteriovenus hemofiltration
CB	carbenicillin catheterized bladder ceased breathing cesarean birth chronic bronchitis Code Blue (emergency medicine) color blind coronary bypass
C & B	chair and bed (rest) crown and bridge (dentistry)
CBA	chronic bronchitis and asthma cost benefit analysis

CBBB	complete bundle branch block
CBC	complete blood count
CBD	closed bladder drainage common bile duct
CBE	clinical breast examination congenital biliary ectasia
CBF	cerebral blood flow coronary blood flow
CBG	capillary blood glucose cortisol-binding globulin
CBI	continuous bladder irrigation
CBP	chronic benign pain complete breech presentation (obstetrics)
CBR	complete bed rest crude birth rate
$\mathbf{C_{BR}}$	bilirubin clearance
CBS	chronic brain syndrome
CBT	carotid body tumor computed body tomography
CBV	catheter balloon valvuloplasty central blood volume circulating blood volume
CBVD	cerebrovascular disease
CC	cardiac cycle cervical collar chest compression

CC *(cont)*	circulatory collapse clindamycin clinical course closing capacity continuing care cord compression costochondral cradle cap creatinine clearance critical care critical condition current complaints
C/C	chief complaint
cc	cubic centimeter with correction (eye examination)
C & C	confirmed and compatible cold and clammy
CCA	cholecystic atony circumflex coronary artery common carotid artery
CC & A	cardiac catheterization and angiography
CCABA	cold, cough, allergy, bronchodilator, antiasthmatic
CCB	calcium channel blocker
CCBV	central circulating blood volume
CCC	care-cure coordination child care clinic
CCCR	closed chest cardiac resuscitation
CCD	calcified cellular debris

CCD *(cont)* charge-coupled device

CCE clubbing, cyanosis, edema

CCI chronic coronary insufficiency

CCK cholecystokinin

CCL critical carbohydrate level

CCM chronic cystic mastitis
congestive cardiomyopathy
critical care medicine

CCMSU clean catch midstream urine

CCN community care network
critical care nursing

CcO_2 oxygen content of pulmonary end-capillary blood

CCP chronic calcifying pancreatitis

CCPD continuous cycled peritoneal dialysis

CCR complete continuous remission

C_{cr} creatinine clearance

CCRC continuing care retirement community

CCRU critical care recovery unit

CCS Cheshire cat syndrome (symptoms without findings)
concentration camp syndrome
critical care services

CCSCS central cervical spinal cord syndrome

CCT	carotid compression tomography coronary care team
CCTD	craniocarpotarsal dystrophy
CCU	coronary care unit critical care unit
CCUA	clean catch urinalysis
CCV	canine coronavirus
CCVD	chronic cerebrovascular disease
CCW	counterclockwise
Ccw	chest wall compliance
CCX	complications
CD	cadaver donor (transplantations) cardiac disease cardiac dullness cardiovascular disease caudal cesarean delivery common duct communicable disease conjugata diagonalis (pelvic measurement) constant drainage convulsive disorder curative dose current diagnosis cystic duct
C/d	cigarettes per day
C & D	curettage and desiccation cystoscopy and dilatation

CDAC	complement-dependent antibody-mediated cytotoxicity
C & DB	cough and deep breath
CDC	cardiac decompensation Centers for Disease Control chronic degenerative disease
CDE	chlordiazepoxide (Librium) common duct exploration
CDEF	chemically defined enteral feeding
CDGD	constitutional delay in growth and development
CDGN	chronic diffuse glomerulonephritis
CDH	chronic daily headache congenital diaphragmatic hernia congenital dislocation of hip
CDI	Children's Depression Inventory clam digger's itch (dermatology)
CDILD	chronic diffuse interstitial lung disease
CDM	clinical decision making
CDN	carbon dioxide narcosis
CDP	comprehensive discharge planning continuous distending pressure cytidine diphosphate
CDR	chronologic drinking review
CDS	cardiovascular surgery congenital dermal sinus

CDT	carbon dioxide therapy
CDU	chemical dependency unit
C_{dyn}	dynamic compliance (of lung)
CE	cardiac emergency cardiac enlargement cerebral edema cholesterol esters contrast enema corrective exercise
CEA	carcinoembryonic antigen carotid endarterectomy cost-effectiveness analysis
CEBV	chronic Epstein Barr virus
CEC	corneal endothelial cell
CECT	contrast-enhanced computed tomography (scanning)
CED	chondroectodermal dysplasia compulsive eating disorder congenital ectodermal defect
CEF	chick embryo fibroblast (vaccine)
CEG	cyberencephalography chronic erosive gastritis
CEI	continuous extravascular infusion
CEM	continuous electrocardiographic monitoring
CEOM	chronic exudative otitis media

CEP	cortical evoked potential (neurology) counterelectrophoresis (test)
ceph floc	cephalin flocculation
CER	central episiotomy and repair conditioned emotional response
CES	clitoral engorgement syndrome
CET	cuffed endotracheal tube
CF	cancer-free cardiac failure Causcasian female central field (eye examination) cephalothin Christmas factor (blood) complement fixation contractile force cough fracture count fingers (eye examination) cystic fibrosis
cf	compare (Latin: *confer*)
CFA	common femoral artery complement-fixing antibody craniofacial abnormality
cfc	colony-forming cell
CFD	craniofacial dysostosis
CFF	critical fusion frequency (test)
CFG	chronic familial granulomatosis
CFI	cardiac function index complement fixation inhibition (test)

CFIDS	chronic fatigue immune deficiency syndrome
CFM	craniofacial microsomia
CFNS	chills, fever, night sweats
CFP	chronic false positive (test)
CFS	chronic fatigue syndrome
CFT	complement fixation test
cfu	colony-forming unit (microbiology)
CG	cardio-green (dye) cholecystogram chorionic gonadotropin colloidal gold (laboratory/serology) control group
CGA	comprehensive geriatric assessment
CGB	chronic gastrointestinal bleeding
CGD	chromosomal gonadal dysgenesis chronic granulomatous disease
CGH	chorionic gonadotropic hormone comparative genome hybridization
CGL	chronic granulocytic leukemia
CGM	central gray matter
CGN	chronic glomerulonephritis
CGP	chorionic growth hormone prolactin
CGPF	cell-growth potentiating factor

CGRP	calcitonin gene-related peptide
CGS	catgut suture centimeter-gram-second
CGT	chorionic gonadotropin
CGTT	cortisone-glucose tolerance test
CH	case history cluster headache Community Health convalescence hospital conversion hysteria crown-heel (length of fetus)
ch	chest chief child chronic
CHA	chronic hemolytic anemia congenital hypoplastic anemia
CHAS	continuous hepatic artery syndrome
CHB	complete heart block (ECG)
CHC	community health center
CHD	childhood disease congenital heart disease coronary heart disease
CHE	cholinesterase
CHF	congestive heart failure
CHFV	combined-high frequency ventilation

CHH	cartilage-hair hypoplasia
CHI	closed head injury creatinine height index
CHIP	comprehensive health insurance plan
CHL	chloramphenicol
CHMD	clinical hyaline membrane disease
CHN	community health nurse
CHO	carbohydrate (diet order)
chol	cholesterol (laboratory/chemistry)
CHOP	cyclophosphamide, hydroxydaunomycin oncovin, prednisone
CHP	child psychiatry comprehensive health plan
chpx	chicken pox
chr	chronic
CHS	compression hip screw (orthopedics)
CHT	congenital hypothyroidism
CI	cardiac index cerebral infarction clinical investigation color index complete iridectomy coronary insufficiency crystalline insulin
Ci	Curie (measurement of activity)

CIB	Carnation Instant Breakfast
CIBD	chronic inflammatory bowel disease
CIBP	chronic intractable benign pain
CICE	combined intracapsular cataract extraction
CICS	cardioinhibitory carotid sinus
CICU	coronary intensive care unit
CID	combined immunodeficiency disease cytomegalic inclusion disease
CIDS	cellular immune deficiency syndrome continuous insulin delivery system
CIEP	counterimmunoelectrophoresis
CIF	claims inquiry form cloning inhibition factor
cig	cigarettes
CIH	carbohydrate-induced hyperglycemia
CIHD	chronic ischemic heart disease
CIL	center for independent living
CIM	changes in menses cortical induction of movement
CIN	cervical intraepithelial neoplasia
C_{in}	insulin clearance
CIOF	chromosomally incompetent ovarian failure

CIOH	chronic idiopathic orthostatic hypotension
CIPF	clinical illness promotion factor
CIPN	chronic idiopathic peripheral neuropathy
circ	circular circulation circumcision
circ & sen	circulation and sensation
CIRR	cirrhosis
CIS	carcinoma in situ clinical information system
CIT	crisis intervention therapy
CIU	chronic idiopathic urticaria
CIV	continuous intravenous (infusion)
CIVII	continuous intravenous insulin infusion
CJD	Creutzfeldt-Jakob disease
CJS	costochondral junction syndrome
CK	creatine kinase (laboratory/chemistry)
ck	check
CL	chest and left arm (ECG lead) cholesterol-lecithin (test) cirrhosis of the liver clot lysis colistin (on culture and sensitivity reports) corpus luteum critical list

Cl	chloride (laboratory/chemistry) clavicle clinic Clostridium (on bacteriology reports)
C_L	lung compliance
cl	clear
CLAH	congenital lipoid adrenal hyperplasia
CLAS	congenital localized absence of skin
CLBBB	complete left bundle branch block
CL/CP	cleft lip/cleft palate
CLD	chronic liver disease chronic lung disease
cldy	cloudy
CLE	centrilobular emphysema
CLH	chronic lobular hepatitis congenital lipoid hyperplasia
CLHN	centrilobular hepatic necrosis
clin	clinical
CLL	cholesterol-lowering lipid chronic lymphocytic leukemia
CLMB	cutaneous lineal melanoblastosis
CLN	computer liaison nurse
CLO	cyclooxygenase

CLP	cleft lip-palate clinical pathology
CLT	clot-lysis time
clysis	hypodermoclysis (procedure/fluid infusion)
CM	case manager Caucasian male cervical mucus cochlear microphonics common migraine congenital malformation contrast media (dye) costal margin
C/M	counts per minute
cm	centimeter tomorrow morning (Latin: *cras mane*)
cm^2	square centimeter
cm^3	cubic centimeter
CMA	certified medical assistant chronic metabolic acidosis
CMBBT	cervical mucus basal body temperature
CMC	carboxymethyl cellulose care management continuity carpometacarpal (joint)
CMCC	chronic mucocutaneous candidiasis
CMD	childhood muscular dystrophy
CME	continuing medical education crude marijuana extract

CMF	cyclophosphamide, methotrexate, 5-fluorouracil (chemotherapy)
CMG	cystometrogram
CMGN	chronic membranous glomerulonephritis
CMH	congenital malformation of the heart
CMHC	Community Mental Health Center
CMI	care management integration cell-mediated immunity computerized medical information Cornell Medical Index
CMID	cytomegalic inclusion disease
c/min	cycles per minute
CMIR	cell-mediated immune response
CMIT	Current Medical Information and Terminology
CMJ	carpometacarpal joint
CML	cell-mediated lympholysis chronic myelogenous leukemia
CMM	cerebellomedullary malformation cutaneous malignant melanoma
CMN	cystic medial necrosis
CMO	cardiac minute output comfort measures only
C-MOPP	cyclophosphamide, mechlorethamine, oncovin, procarbazine, prednisone

CMP	cardiomyopathy comprehensive medical plan
CMR	cerebral metabolic rate
CMS	central material supply chronic mycelial stomatitis costal margin syndrome
CMT	Certified Medical Transcriptionist Charcot-Marie-Tooth (syndrome)
CMV	continuous mechanical ventilation cytomegalovirus
CMVS	culture mid-void specimen
CN	charge nurse clinical nurse cranial nerve
CNA	Certified Nurse Assistant chart not available
CND	cause not determined congenital neuromuscular disorder
CNDO	complete neglect of differential overlap
CNE	chronic nervous exhaustion could not establish
CNH	community nursing home
CNL	cardiolipin natural lecithin community nursing liaison
CNM	Certified Nurse Midwife
CNOR	Certified Nurse, Operating Room

CNP	constant negative pressure
CNPAP	continuous nasal positive airway pressure
CNR	coronary nodal rhythm
CNS	central nervous system clinical nurse specialist computerized notation system
CNSD	chronic nonspecific diarrhea (toddler diarrhea)
CNSLD	chronic nonspecific lung disease
CNT	could not test
CNV	conduction nerve velocity (neurologic test)
CO	carbon monoxide cardiac output castor oil central obesity co-insurance continuous observation corneal opacity coronary occlusion court order
c/o	check out complains of
^{60}CO	radioactive cobalt (nuclear medicine)
CO_2	carbon dioxide
COA	child of alcoholic coarctation of aorta
CoA	coenzyme A

COAD	chronic obstructive airway disease
coag	coagulase (on bacteriology reports) coagulation
coag T	coagulation time
COAP	cyclophosphamide, oncovin, cytosine, arabinoside, prednisone
COBT	chronic obstruction of biliary tract
COC	certificate of coverage
CO_2 comb	carbon dioxide combining power
CO_2 cont	carbon dioxide content
COD	cause of death chemical oxygen demand condition on discharge
CODM	craniooculoorbital dysraphia-meningocele
CODO	codocytes
Cod SO_4	codeine sulfate
COE	court-ordered examination
COG	closed angle glaucoma
COGN	cognition
COGTT	cortisone-primed oral glucose tolerance test
COH	carbohydrate control of hemorrhage

COHb	carboxyhemoglobin (laboratory/chemistry)
COI	certificate of insurance
COL	cost of living
col	colony (on culture reports) colored
COLD	chronic obstructive lung disease
cold agg	cold agglutinin
COM	cyclophosphamide, oncovin, methotrexate (chemotherapy)
comm	communicable
comp	compensated (heart disease) compensation (case) complaint complete complication composition compound
COMS	chronic organic mental syndrome
conc	concentration
cond	condition conduction
cont	containing contents continue contusion
contra	contraindicated

conv convalescent

COOD chronic obstructive outflow disease

COP capillary osmotic pressure

COPD chronic obstructive pulmonary disease

COPE chronic obstructive pulmonary emphysema
cyclophosphamide, oncovin, platinol, etophoside (chemotherapy)

COPP cyclophosphamide, oncovin, procarbazine, prednisone (chemotherapy)

COPU cutaneous oropharyngeal ulceration

COR conditioned orientation response

CORLA clusters of radiolucent areas (radiology)

cort cortex
cortical
cortisone

COS change of shift (hospital)
Chief of Staff

COTA Certified Occupational Therapy Assistant

CP canal paresis
capillary pressure
cerebral palsy
chemically pure
chest pain
chickenpox
chronic pain
chronic pyelonephritis
cleft palate
closing pressure (spinal tap)

CP *(cont)*	combining power complete physical convenience package coproporphyrin cornual pregnancy coronal plane cor pulmonale creatine phosphate
C & P	complete and pushing cystoscopy and panendoscopy
CPA	cardiopulmonary arrest carotid phonoangiography cerebellar pontine angle conditioned play audiometry
c:pa	crown to pubic arch ratio
$\mathbf{C_{pah}}$	para-aminohippurate clearance
CPAP	continuous positive airway pressure
CPB	cardiopulmonary bypass competitive protein binding (assay)
CPBS	cardiopulmonary bypass surgery
CPC	chronic passive congestion clinicopathologic correlation community psychiatric center
CP & C	cast post and core (dentistry)
CPD	calcium pyrophosphate dihydrate (crystals) cephalopelvic disproportion congenital polycystic disease
Cpd E	cortisone (Compound E)

Cpd F	hydrocortisone (Compound F)
CPE	cardiogenic pulmonary edema chronic pulmonary emphysema
CPF	clot-promoting factor
CPG	craniopharyngioma
CPGN	chronic progressive glomerulonephritis
CPI	congenital pain indifference coronary prognostic index cost-patient index
CPID	chronic pelvic inflammatory disease
CPI-MCS	consumer price index — medical care services
CPK	creatine phosphokinase (same as CK)
cpm	counts per minute
CPN	chronic pyelonephritis
CPNC	chronic progressive nonhereditary chorea
CPP	cerebral perfusion pressure chronic pelvic pain
CPPB	continuous positive pressure breathing
CP & PD	chest percussion and postural drainage
CPPV	continuous positive pressure ventilation
CPR	cardiopulmonary resuscitation computerized patient records cortisol production rate

CPRD chronic progressive renal disease

CPRS Children's Psychiatric Rating Scale

CPS clinical performance score

cps cycles per second

CPT carotid pulse tracing
chest physiotherapy (respiratory therapy)

CPU central processing unit

CPX complete physical examination

CPZ chlorpromazine (Thorazine)

C & Q chloroquine and quinine

CQI continuous quality improvement

CR cardiorespiratory
chest and right arm (ECG lead)
clot retraction
colon resection
complete remission
conditioned reflex
controlled release
conversion reaction (psychiatry)
corneal reflex
crown-rump (length of fetus)

Cr cranial
creatine
Cryptococcus (on bacteriology reports)

^{51}Cr radioactive chromium (nuclear medicine)

CRA central retinal artery

CRAA cerebroretinal arteriovenous aneurysm

CRAMS circulation, respiration, abdomen, motor, speech

CRAO central retinal artery occlusion (eye examination)

CRBBB complete right bundle branch block (ECG)

CRC colorectal cancer
crisis resolution center (psychiatry)

CRD chronic renal disease
chronic respiratory disease
contractile ring dysphagia
crown-rump distance

CRE cumulative radiation effect

creat creatinine (laboratory/chemistry)

CREST calcinosis cutis, Raynaud's phenomenon, esophageal dysfunction hypermotility, sclerodactyly, telangiectasia (syndrome)

CRF case report form
chronic renal failure

CRG cardiorespirogram

CRH corticotropin-releasing hormone

CRI Cardiac Risk Index
chronic renal insufficiency

CRIE crossed radioimmunoelectrophoresis

crit critical

CRL	Certified Record Librarian crown-rump length
CRM	cross-reacting material
Crn	crown (dentistry)
cRNA	chromosomal ribonucleic acid
CRNP	Certified Registered Nurse Practitioner
CRP	colorectal polyps confluent reticular papillomatosis C-reactive protein (laboratory/hematology)
CrP	creatine phosphate
CRRT	Certified Respiratory Therapy Technician
CRS	Chinese restaurant syndrome (glutamic acid toxicity) colorectal surgery
CRST	calcinosis, Raynaud's phenomenon, sclerodactyly and telangiectasia (syndrome)
CRT	cardiac resuscitation team cathode ray tube complex reaction time computed renal tomography
crt	hematocrit
CRTX	cast removed, take to x-ray
CRV	central retinal vein
CRVO	central retinal vein occlusion
crys	crystalline

CS	cardiogenic shock carotid sinus Central Service (Central Supply) cerebrospinal (fluid) cesarean section chronic schizophrenia clinical stage (tumor classification) completed suicide concentrated strength (drugs) conditioned stimulus congenital syphilis conscious coronal suture coronary sinus corpus striatum corticosteroid cromolyn sodium
C_s	static compliance (lungs)
cs	case conscious
C & S	conjunctiva and sclera (eye examination) culture and sensitivity
CSA	central sleep apnea cross-sectional area
CSB	chemical stimulation of the brain
CSBF	coronary sinus blood flow
CSBO	complete small bowel obstruction
CSC	cardiac sphincter chalasia cornea, sclera, conjunctiva crankcase spool catheter
CSCT	comprehensive support care team

CSD celiac sprue disease
cervical spine dislocation
chemical sensitivity disorder

CS & D cleaned, sutured and dressed

CSE cross-section echocardiography

CSF cerebrospinal fluid
colony-stimulating factor

CSG chronic simple glaucoma

CSH chronic subdural hematoma
congenital subluxation of the hip

CSHEP constriction, sclerosis, hemorrhage, exudate, papilledema

CSI cholesterol saturation index
continuous subcutaneous insulin (infusion)

CSM carotid sinus massage (cardiology)
cerebrospinal meningitis

CSN carotid sinus nerve

CSOM chronic serous otitis media

CSP carotid sinus pressure

CSR central serous retinopathy
Central Supply Room
Cheyne-Stokes respiration
corrected sedimentation rate
cortisol secretion rate

CSS carotid sinus stimulation
central sterile supply
chewing, sucking, swallowing

CSSD	corticostriatal spinal degeneration
CST	cardiac stress test cavernous sinus thrombosis cognitive skill training contraction stress test convulsive shock therapy
CSU	cardiac surveillance unit catheter specimen of urine
CSUF	continuous slow ultrafiltration
CT	carotid tracing (procedure/cardiology) carpal tunnel (syndrome) cerebral thrombosis cervical traction chemotherapy chest tube chlorothiazide (diuretic) circulation time (procedure/cardiology) clotting time (laboratory/hematology) coagulation time (laboratory/hematology) coated tablet cognitive therapy computerized tomography (procedure/x-ray) connective tissue contraction time (obstetrics) Coomb's test (laboratory/blood bank) corneal transplant coronary thrombosis cover test
C/T	compression-traction ratio
ct	count
CTA	chemotactic activity clear to auscultation cytoplasmic tubular aggregates

CTA *(cont)*	cytotoxic assay
CTB	ceased to breathe
CTC	congenital thrombocytopenia
CTCL	cutaneous T-cell lymphoma
CTD	carpal tunnel decompression chest tube drainage connective tissue disease
CT & DB	cough, turn and deep breathe
CTDW	continues to do well
CTE	congenital telangiectatic erythema
CTF	cancer therapy facility contrast transfer function
C/TG	cholesterol-triglyceride ratio
CTL	cytotoxic T-lymphocyte
CTP	comprehensive treatment plan
CTR	cardiothoracic ratio
CTS	carpal tunnel syndrome computerized tomographic scan
CTSP	called to see patient
CTT	computed transaxial tomography
CTU	cardiothoracic unit
CTX	cervical traction

CTx	cardiac transplantation
CTXN	contraction (obstetrics)
CTZ	chemoreceptor trigger zone chlorothiazide
CU	cause unknown control unit Couvelaire uterus
Cu	copper
C_u	urea clearance (renal function test)
CUC	chronic ulcerative colitis
CUD	cause undetermined congenital urinary (tract) deformities
CUG	cystourethrogram (procedure/urology)
CUHB	chronic unconjugated hyperbilirubinemia
cu mm	cubic millimeter
CUPP	conservative uvulopalatoplasty
CUR	cystourethrocele
CUS	cartoid ultrasound (procedure/neurology)
CV	cardiovascular cell volume central venous (pressure) cerebrovascular closing volume (in pulmonary function test reports) color vision (eye examination) coma vigil

CV *(cont)*	conduction velocity corpuscular volume (red blood cells)
c/v	cupping and vibrating (pulmonary physiotherapy)
CVA	cardiovascular accident cerebrovascular accident (stroke) costovertebral angle
CVC	central venous catheter
CVCT	cardiovascular computerized tomography
CVD	cardiovascular disease cerebrovascular disease collagen vascular disease
cvd	curved
CVE	cerebrovascular episode
CVF	central visual field
CVG	contrast ventriculography coronary vein graft (operation/cardiac)
CVI	cerebrovascular insufficiency continuous venous infusion
CVM	cardiovascular monitor
CVN	central venous nutrient
CVO	central vein occlusion conjugate diameter of pelvic inlet (Latin: *conjugata vera obstetrica*)
C_vO_2	mixed venous oxygen content

CVP	cardiac valve pressure central venous pressure
CVPP	cyclophosphamide, vincristine, prednisone, procarbazine (chemotherapy)
CVR	cardiovascular-respiratory (system) cerebrovascular resistance
CVRD	cardiovascular renal disease
CVS	cardiovascular surgery cardiovascular system chorionic villi sampling (procedure/gynecology) clean-voided specimen (procedure/urine culture)
CVUG	cystoscopy and voiding urethrogram
CW	cardiac work case worker chest wall clockwise crutch walking
cw	cell wall
CWD	continuous-wave Doppler (radiology)
CWI	cardiac work index
CWS	cold water soluble cotton-wool spots (ophthalmology)
CX	chest x-ray craniohypophyseal xanthoma
Cx	cancel

cx	cervix convex
CxMT	cervical motion tenderness (gynecology)
cyclo	cyclopropane (anesthetic)
CYL	casein yeast lactate
CYS	cystoscopy (procedure/urology)
CZI	crystalline zinc insulin

D

D	daughter deceased diagnosis diarrhea diopter (eye examination) disease dispense (on prescriptions) divorced donor dorsal (spines)
d	day decreased density diameter diastolic distal dose duration right (Latin: *dextro*)
D_1 to D_{12}	dorsal vertebrae (1 through 12)
DA	degenerative arthritis delayed action (drugs) dental assistant developmental age diabetic acidosis direct admission direct agglutination disability assistance dopamine ductus arteriosus
D/A	date of admission
DAB	days after birth

DAD	dispense as directed
DAEM	disseminated acute encephalomyelitis
DAH	disordered action of the heart
DAMA	discharged against medical advice
DAP	Draw-a-Person Test (psychiatry)
DAPT	direct agglutination pregnancy test
DAR	daily affective rhythm
DARP	drug abuse rehabilitation program
DAS	Dyadic Adjustment Scale (psychiatry)
DAT	delayed action tablet dementia of Alzheimer's type diet as tolerated (diet order) diphtheria antitoxin direct antiglobulin test
dAT	direct agglutination test
DAW	dispense as written (on prescriptions)
DB	date of birth deep breath
Db	diabetic
db	decibel
DB & C	deep breath and cough
DBCL	dilute blood clot lysis
DBE	deep breathing exercise

DBE *(cont)*	diffuse bone endothelioma
DBF	disturbed bowel function
DBI	development at birth index
DBM	diabetic management
DBN	downbeat nystagmus (ophthalmology)
DBP	diastolic blood pressure double breech presentation (obstetrics)
DBS	despeciated bovine serum diminished breath sounds
DBW	desirable body weight
DC	daily census diabetic coma diagnostic code (on records) diagonal conjugate diffusing capacity donor cells
D/C	diarrhea/constipation discharge discontinue
D & C	dilation and curettage (operation/gynecology)
DCA	desoxycorticosterone acetate (medication order) directional coronary arterectomy
DCABG	double coronary artery bypass graft
DCB	dilutional cardiopulmonary bypass

DCBE	double contrast barium enema (procedure/x-ray)
DCC	day care center
DCc	double concave (ophthalmology)
DCF	day care facility direct centrifugal flotation
DCG	dacryocystography (procedure/ophthalmology) dynamic electrocardiography (procedure/cardiology)
DCH	delayed cutaneous hypersensitivity
DCI	duplicate coverage inquiry
DCIS	ductal carcinoma in situ (mammography finding)
DCN	delayed conditioned necrolysis
D_{co}	diffusing capacity for carbon monoxide (pulmonary function test)
DCP	discharge plan
DCR	dacryocystorhinostomy direct cortical response
DCSA	double contrast shoulder arthrography
DCT	direct Coomb's test (laboratory/blood bank) distal convoluted tubule (of kidney)
DCTM	delay computer tomographic myelography
DCU	diabetes care unit

DCx	double convex (ophthalmology)
DD	dangerous drug degenerative disease dependent drainage developmentally disadvantaged died of the disease differential diagnosis disc diameter (eye examination) double diffusion (test) double dose dry dressing
D & D	diarrhea and dehydration
DDB	donor directed blood
ddC	dideoxycytidine (AIDS treatment drug)
DDD	degenerative disc disease
DDI	dressing dry and intact
ddI	dideoxyinosine (AIDS treatment drug)
DDR	discharged during referral
DDRA	dead despite resuscitation attempt
DDS	directional Doppler sonography Doctor of Dental Surgery
DDST	Denver Developmental Screening Test (pediatrics)
DDT	dichlorodiphenyltrichloroethane
DDx	differential diagnosis
DE	drug equivalent

DE *(cont)*	dose evaluation
2-DE	two-dimensional echocardiogram
D & E	dilation and evacuation
DEA#	Drug Enforcement Administration number (physician's narcotic number)
deb	debridement
decd	deceased
decomp	decompensated (heart disease) decomposed
decr	decreased
DED	date of expected delivery (obstetrics) delayed erythema dose (radiology)
DEF	decayed, extracted, filled (teeth)
def	defecation deficient definite definition
defic	deficiency deficit
deg	degeneration degree
degen	degeneration
Dem	Demerol (meperidine hydrochloride)
DEP	diatomaceous earth pneumoconiosis

depr	depression
DER	dermatology died in emergency room
deriv	derivative
DES	diethylstilbestrol diffuse esophageal spasm
desat	desaturated
desc	descending
DEUC	direct electronic urethrocystometry
DEV	duck embryo vaccine
Dev	deviation
devel	development
DEXA	dual energy x-ray absorptiometry
DF	decayed and filled (teeth) diabetic father dietary fiber digital fluoroscopy disseminated foci dorsiflexion
DFA	diet for age direct fluorescent antibody (technique)
DFI	darkfield illumination disease free interval
DFMC	daily fetal movement count
DFP	diastolic filling period (cardiology)

DFR	dialysate filtration rate
DFS	disease-free survival
DFT_4	dialyzable free thyroxine (laboratory/endocrinology)
DFU	dead fetus in utero
DG	diagnosis diastolic gallop
DGA	dermatoglyphic alteration
DGI	deoxyglucose imaging disseminated gonococcal infection
DGM	ductal glandular mastectomy
dgm	decigram (measurement)
DGR	Dacron graft replacement
DGS	diabetic glomerulosclerosis
DH	delayed hypersensitivity dental hygiene developmental history diaphragmatic hernia drug hypersensitivity
DHE	dihydroergotamine
DHEA	dihydroepiandrosterone
DHN	dissociative hysterical neurosis
DHR	delayed hypersensitivity reaction
DHS	duration of hospital stay

DHS *(cont)*	dynamic hip screw
D/5 HS	5% dextrose in Hartman's solution (intravenous solution)
DHSM	dihydrostreptomycin (on culture and sensitivity reports)
DHT	dihydrotachysterol
DI	diabetes insipidus diagnostic imaging disability insurance drug interactions
D & I	debridement and irrigation
DIA	diabetes
diab	diabetic
diag	diagnostic diagonal
diam	diameter
diath	diathermy (physical therapy)
DIB	disability insurance benefit
DIC	diffuse intravascular coagulation disseminated intravascular coagulation drug information center
DID	double immunodiffusion
DIE	direct injection enthalpimetry
DIF	diffuse interstitial fibrosis direct immunofluorescence (test)

diff	difference differential blood count (laboratory/hematology)
DIG	digoxin (medication order)
dig	digitalis (medication order) digitate
Dil	Dilantin (diphenylhydantoin)
dil	dilute
dilat	dilatation
DILD	diffuse infiltrative lung disease
DILE	drug-induced lupus erythematosis
dim	diminished
dim 1/2	diminish by half (medication order)
DIP	desquamative interstitial pneumonia drip infusion pyelogram
Dip	Dipaxin (diphenadione)
DIPC	diffuse interstitial pulmonary calcification
diph	diphtheria
diph/tet	diphtheria-tetanus (toxoid) (medication order)
diph tox	diphtheria toxoid (medication order)
diph tox AP	diphtheria toxoid-alum precipitated (medication order)

DIPJ	distal interphalangeal joint
DIR	delivered in room
Dir	director
dir	direct
dis	disabled disease
disc	discontinue
disch	discharge
DISH	diffuse idiopathic skeletal hyperostosis
disloc	dislocation
dism	dismissed
disp	dispense (medication orders/prescriptions)
dissd	dissolved
dissem	disseminated
dist	distance distill disturbance
DIT	diet-induced thermogenesis
div	divergence divide
DIVA	digital intravenous angiography
diz	dizygotic

DJD	degenerative joint disease
DJS	Dubin-Johnson syndrome
Dk	diffusion coefficient (pulmonary medicine)
dk	dark
DKA	diabetic ketoacidosis
DKB	deep knee bends
DL	danger list developmental level direct laryngoscopy distolingual (dentistry)
dl	deciliter
D_L	diffusing capacity of the lung
DL Ab	Donath-Landsteiner antibody (hemolysis) (laboratory/blood bank)
D_LCO	diffusing capacity of the lung for carbon monoxide
DLE	discoid lupus erythematosus disseminated lupus erythematosus
DLG	disseminated lipogranulomatosis
DLH	dislocated hip
D_5LR	5% dextrose in lactated Ringer's (intravenous solution)
DM	diabetes mellitus diabetic mother diastolic murmur

Dm	diffusing capacity of alveolar membrane
DMA	directed memory access (psychiatry)
DMARD	disease-modifying antirheumatic drug
DMAT	disaster medical assistance team
DMC	direct microscopic count
DMCT	demethylchlortetracycline
DMD	disciform macular degeneration distal muscular dystrophy Doctor of Medical Dentistry
DME	Director of Medical Education durable medical equipment
DMF	decayed, missing, filled (teeth)
DMI	diaphragmatic myocardial infarction
DML	diffuse mixed lymphoma
DMP	dermatopathology
DMPA	durable medical power of attorney
DMS	delayed muscle soreness dermatomyositis
DMSO	dimethylsulfoxide
DMX	diathermy, massage, exercise (physical therapy)
DN	diabetic neuropathy dicrotic notch down

DN *(cont)*	dysplastic nevi (dermatology)
DNA	deoxyribonucleic acid do not administer
DNase	deoxyribonuclease
DNC	do not close (surgery)
DND	died a natural death
DNI	do not intubate
DNKA	did not keep appointment
DNP	do not publish
DNR	do not resuscitate
DNS	deviated nasal septum did not show do not substitute dysplastic nevus syndrome (dermatology)
D5/NSS	5% dextrose in normal saline solution (intravenous solution)
DNT	did not test do not treat
dnt	do not take
DO	diastolic overload diet order dissolved oxygen Doctor of Osteopathy
D/O	disorder
d/o	died of

DOA	date of arrival dead on arrival
DOB	date of birth
DOC	died of other causes drug of choice
DOCA	desoxycorticosterone acetate (medication order)
DOD	date of death date of discharge day of delivery dead of disease
DOE	date of examination degree of exercise dyspnea on exertion
DOI	date of injury
DON	Director of Nursing
DOP	dopamine
DOPS	diffusion obstructive pulmonary syndrome
DORx	date of treatment
DOS	day of surgery
DOT	died on operating table Doppler ophthalmic test
DOU	direct observation unit
DOV	discharged on visit
DOX	doxorubicin

DP	desquamative pneumonia diastolic pressure diffuse pressure direct puncture directional preponderance distal phalanx (orthopedics) donor plasma dorsalis pedis (pulse) double pneumonia
DPA	dextroposition of aorta dual photon absorptiometry
DPC	delayed primary closure direct patient care
DPD	diffuse pulmonary disease
dp/dt	ratio of change of ventricular pressure to change of time
DPG	displacement placentogram (radiology)
DPH	diphenylhydantoin (Dilantin)
DPIF	Drug Product Information File
dpm	disintegrations per minute (nuclear medicine)
DPM	Doctor of Podiatric Medicine
DPN	dermatopolyneuritis
DPOAE	distortion product otoacoustic emission
DPP	documented poor prognosis
DPT	diabetic pseudotabes

DPT *(cont)*	diphtheria, pertussis, tetanus (vaccine) (medication order)
DPTI	diastolic pressure-time index
DQ	developmental quotient (pediatrics)
DQF	double quotidian fever
DR	delivery room diabetic retinopathy diagnostic radiology diastolic rumble dorsal root (spinal nerves)
dr	dram dressing
DRA	drug-related admission
DRAD	dwarfism with retinal atrophy and deafness
DRE	digital rectal examination
DRF	daily replacement factor
DRG	diagnosis related group dorsal root ganglion
D(Rh_o)	blood antigen
DRQ	discomfort relief quotient
DS	dead air space (pulmonary function test) dental surgery dextran sulfate dextrose saline dilute strength (of solution) dissolved solids

DS *(cont)*	donor serum Down's syndrome dry swallow (medication order) duration of systole
D/S	dextrose in saline
D5/S	5% dextrose in saline
DSA	digital subtraction angiogram (procedure/cardiology)
DSD	discharge summary dictated dry sterile dressing
DSE	digital subtraction echocardiogram
dsg	dressing
DSI	digital subtraction imaging (cardiology)
DSM-IV	Diagnostic and Statistical Manual of Mental Disorders, 4th Edition
DSP	decreased sensory perception
DSR	diffuse syncytial reticulosarcoma
DSS	dermatitis schistosomiasis disability status scale
DST	desensitization test (allergy) dexamethasone suppression test dihydrostreptomycin (on culture and sensitivity reports) dural sinus thrombosis
DSVP	downstream venous pressure

DT	dental technician diphtheria-tetanus (toxoid) distance test (hearing) double tachycardia
DTA	displacement threshold acuity
DTC	day treatment center
DTH	delayed-type hypersensitivity
DTO	deodorized tincture of opium
DTP	diphtheria, tetanus, pertussis (vaccine) distal tingling on percussion
DTR	deep tendon reflex
DT's	delirium tremens
DTT	diphtheria-tetanus toxoid disaccharide tolerance test (diagnostic procedure)
DTX	detoxification
DTx	diphtheria toxoid
DTx-AP	diphtheria toxoid-alum precipitated
DU	decubitus ulcer diabetic urine diagnosis undetermined duodenal ulcer
D & U	diffuse and undifferentiated
DUB	dysfunctional uterine bleeding
DUG	drug use guidelines

DUI	driving under influence (of alcohol or drugs)
DUL	diffuse undifferentiated lymphoma
DuMD	Duchenne's muscular dystrophy
DUR	drug usage review
DUS	Doppler ultrasound stethoscope
DV	dilute volume (of solution) double vision
D & V	diarrhea and vomiting
DVA	distance visual acuity (eye examination)
DVD	dissociated vertical divergence (ophthalmology)
DVI	digital vascular imaging
DVR	double valve replacement (cardiology)
DVT	deep vein thrombosis
DVVC	direct visualization of vocal cords
DW	distilled water (medication orders/prescriptions) dry weight
D/W	dextrose in water (intravenous solution)
D5/W (D_5W)	5% dextrose in water
DWI	diffusion-weighted imaging driving while intoxicated

DX	dextran
Dx	diagnosis
DXA	dual x-ray absorptiometry
DXM	dexamethasone
DXR	deep x-ray
DXT	deep x-ray therapy
DZ	dizygotic (twins)

E

E	edema emmetropia (eye examination) enema enzyme eosinophil (on white blood count reports) erythromycin (on culture and sensitivity reports) esophoria (eye examination) etiology expired gas (pulmonary function test)
E_1	estrone (laboratory/endocrinology)
E_2	estradiol (17-estradiol) (laboratory/endocrinology
E_3	estriol (laboratory/endocrinology)
E_4	esterol (laboratory/endocrinology)
EA	educational age electroanesthesia emergency area environmental assessment erythrocyte antibody
ea	each
E & A	evaluate and advise
EAA	essential amino acid extrinsic allergic alveolitis
EAB	elective abortion extraanatomic bypass
EABR	electrical-evoked auditory brainstem response

EAC	erythrocyte antibody complement external auditory canal
EACA	epsilon aminocaproic acid (medication order)
EACD	eczematous allergic contact dermatitis
EAE	experimental allergic encephalomyelitis
EAG	electroatriogram
EAHF	eczema, asthma, hay fever
EAL	electronic artificial larynx
EAM	external auditory meatus
EAN	experimental allergic neuritis
EAP	extrinsic allergic pneumonia
EAST	external rotation and abduction stress test (orthopedics)
EAT	ectopic atrial tachycardia
EB	epidermolysis bullosa Epstein-Barr (virus) escape beat
EBBS	equal bilateral breath sounds
EBC	esophageal balloon catheter
EBF	elastic band fixation (fractures) erythroblastosis fetalis
EBL	estimated blood loss (on surgical reports)

EBM	evidence-based medicine expressed breast milk
EBP	erythroblastopenia esophageal balloon procedure estradiol-binding protein
EBS	electronic brain stimulator
EBT	early bedtime
EBV	Epstein-Barr virus
EC	ejection click (cardiology) emergency center enteric-coated (tablets) (medication orders/prescriptions) Escherichia coli (on culture reports) extracapsular extracellular eyes closed
E/C	endoscopy/cystoscopy (urology) estriol-creatinine ratio
ECA	electrocardioanalyser ethacrynic acid
ECAT	emission computerized axial tomography
ECBV	effective circulating blood volume
ECC	edema, clubbing, cyanosis emergency cardiac care endocervical curettage extracorporeal circulation
ECCE	extracapsular cataract extraction (operation/ophthalmology)

ECD	endothelial corneal dystrophy
ECE	endocervical ecchymosis (gynecology)
ECF	epicanthic fold (ophthalmology) extended care facility extracellular fluid
ECFV	extracellular fluid volume
ECG	electrocardiogram (procedure/cardiology)
ECGT	epiphyseal chondromatous giant-cell tumor
ECHO	enterocytopathogenic human orphan (virus)
echo	echocardiogram (procedure/cardiology) echoencephalogram (procedure/neurology)
ECIB	extracorporeal irradiation of blood
ECL	euglobulin clot lysis (laboratory/hematology) extracapillary lesion
ECM	erythema chronicum migrans external cardiac massage extracellular material
ECMO	enterocytopathogenic monkey orphan (virus) extracorporeal membrane oxygenation
ECoG	electrocorticogram (neurology)
E coli	Escherichia coli (laboratory/bacteriology)

ECP eosinophil cationic protein
external counterpulsation

ECPO enterocytopathogenic porcine orphan (virus)

ECS elective cosmetic surgery
electrocerebral silence (brain death)

ECT electroconvulsive therapy
emission computed tomography
enteric-coated tablet (medication orders/prescriptions)

ECU emergency care unit
eternal care unit (morgue)

ECV extracellular volume
extracorporeal volume

ECVE extracellular volume expansion

ECW extracellular water

ED effective dose
electrodialysis
emergency department
epidural
erythema dose
exit dose (radiology)

ED_{50} median effective dose

EDA electrodermal audiometry
end-diastolic area

EDB early dry breakfast

EDC estimated date of confinement

ED & C	electrodessication and curettage
EDD	effective drug duration estimated discharge date expected date of delivery
EDG	electrodermography
EDM	early diastolic murmur electronic daily monitor
EDP	end-diastolic pressure
EDR	effective direct radiation electrodermal response expected death rate
EDS	Ehlers-Danlos syndrome
EDTA	ethylenediaminetetraacetic acid
EDU	eating disorder unit
EDV	end-diastolic volume
EDx	electrodiagnosis
EE	embryo extract end to end (anastomosis) equine encephalitis
E & E	eyes and ears
EEA	electroencephalic audiometry
EEE	eastern equine encephalitis external eye examination
EEG	electroencephalogram (procedure/neurology)

EEGA	electroencephalographic audiometry
EENT	eyes, ears, nose and throat
EEP	end-expiratory pressure (pulmonary function test)
EERP	extended endocardial resection procedure
EF	ectopic focus ejection fraction (heart) elongation factor erythroblastosis fetalis escape focus (cardiology)
EFA	essential fatty acids (laboratory/chemistry)
EFE	endocardial fibroelastosis
EFHC	essential familial hypercholesterolemia
EFHL	essential familial hyperlipemia
EFI	elderly functionally impaired
EFM	electronic fetal monitoring
EFP	emotional facial palsy
EFR	effective filtration rate
EFV	extracellular fluid volume
EFVC	expiratory flow-volume curve (pulmonary function test)
EG	esophagogastrectomy (operation/gastrointestinal) external genitalia

eg	for example (Latin: *exempli gratia*)
EGA	estimated gestational age
EGD	esophagogastroduodenoscopy
EGF	epidermal growth factor
EGG	electrogastrogram (procedure/gastroenterology)
EGL	eosinophilic granuloma of the lung
EGlG	electroglottogram
EGM	electrogustometry
EGS	electric galvanic stimulation (orthopedics)
EGTA	esophageal gastric tube airway
EH	emotionally handicapped enlarged heart essential hypertension
eH	oxidation-reduction potential
EHB	elevate head of bed entrance heart block
EHBF	estimated hepatic blood flow
EHBT	extrahepatic biliary tree
EHC	enterohepatic clearance extended health care
EHH	esophageal hiatal hernia

EHL effective half-life (of radioactive substances)

EHO extrahepatic obstruction

EHP extra high potency

EHPH extrahepatic portal hypertension

EI electrolyte imbalance
enzyme inhibitor

E/I expiration-inspiration ratio (pulmonary function test)

EIA enzyme immunoassay
exercise-induced asthma

EIB exercise-induced bronchospasm

EID electroimmunodiffusion

EIL elective induction of labor

EIN epiphyseal ischemic necrosis

EIP elective interruption of pregnancy
end-inspiratory pressure
extensor indicis proprius

EJ elbow jerk

EJB ectopic junctional beat

EK erythrokinase

EKC epidemic keratoconjunctivitis

EKG electrocardiogram (procedure/cardiology)

EKO	echoencephalogram
EKY	electrokymogram
EL	effective level exercise limit
ELAT	enzyme-linked antiglobulin test
ELB	early light breakfast
elb	elbow
ELF	elective low forceps (delivery)
ELISA	enzyme-linked immunosorbent assay (laboratory procedure)
elix	elixir
ELOS	estimated length of stay
ELP	endogenous lipoid pneumonia
ELT	euglobulin lysis time
EM	ejection murmur electron microscope emergency medicine erythema multiforme erythrocyte mass external monitor
E & M	endocrine and metabolic
Em	emergency emmetropia
EMA	efferent motor aphasia epithelial membrane antigen

EMB	endometrial biopsy
EMC	emergency medical care encephalomyocarditis endometrial curettage
EMDR	eye movement desensitization and reprocessing (antianxiety therapy)
EMF	electromagnetic flowmeter endomyocardial fibrosis erythrocyte maturation factor evaporated milk formula
EMG	electromyogram (procedure/physical medicine)
EMI	electromagnetic interference
EMIC	emergency maternity and infant care
EMIT	enzyme-multiplied immunoassay technique
EMMA	eye movement measuring apparatus
EMR	electromagnetic radiation emergency mechanical restraint endoscopic mucosal resection
EMS	early morning (urine) specimen electronic muscle stimulator emergency medical services eosinophilia-myalgia syndrome
EMT	Emergency Medical Technician
emul	emulsion
EMyB	endomyocardial biopsy

EN	enteral nutrition erythema nodosum
En	enema
ENA	extractable nuclear antigen
ENG	electronystagmogram (procedure/ophthalmology)
ENoG	electroneuronogram
ENR	eosinophilic nonallergic rhinitis
ENT	ears, nose and throat
enz	enzyme
EO	extraocular eyes open
EOA	erosive osteoarthritis esophageal obturator airway examination, opinion and advice
EOAE	evoked otoacoustic emission
EOB	emergency observation bed explanation of benefits
EOC	eosinophil count epiphyseal osteochondritis
EOD	environmental and occupational disorders
eod	every other day
EOG	electrooculogram (procedure/ophthalmology)

EOM	error of measurement extraocular movements extraocular muscles
EOMA	emergency oxygen mask assembly
EOMB	explanation of medical benefits
eos	eosinophils (laboratory/hematology)
EP	ectopic pregnancy electrophoresis emergency procedure enzyme product evoked potentials
EPA	eicosapentaenoic acid evidence of physical abuse
EPC	epilepsy (epilepsia partialis continua)
EPCG	endoscopic pancreatocholangiography
EPEC	enteropathogenic Escherichia coli (laboratory/bacteriology)
EPG	electropneumogram (neurology) exophthalmic goiter
Epi	epinephrine
epith	epithelial
EPM	electronic pacemaker
EPMH	extrapyramidal muscular hypertrophy
EPO	erythropoietin
EPP	equal pressure point

EPR	electron paramagnetic resonance
EPS	early and periodic screening electrical programmed stimulation electrophysiologic studies (cardiology)
EPSP	excitatory postsynaptic potential
EPT	early pregnancy test
EPV	epidemic paralytic vertigo
eq	equivalent
ER	ejection rate emergency room endoplasmic reticulum equivalent roentgen estrogen receptor (test) evoked response extended release (tablet) external rotation (orthopedics)
E&R	equal and regular (ophthalmology)
ERA	evoked response audiometry (procedure/otology)
ERBF	effective renal blood flow
ERC	endoscopic retrograde cholangiography
ERCP	endoscopic retrograde cholangio-pancreatography (procedure/GI)
ERD	evoked response detector external reactive depression
ERG	electroretinogram (procedure/ophthalmology)

ERH experimental renal hypertension

ERIA electroradioimmunoassay

ERL effective refractory length (ophthalmology)

ERNA equilibrium radionuclide angiography (procedure/cardiology)

ERnG echorenogram

ERP effective refractory period
emergency room physician
estrogen receptor protein

ERPD endoscopic retrograde pancreaticoduodenography

ERPF effective renal plasma flow

ERT estrogen replacement therapy

ERV expiratory reserve volume (pulmonary medicine)

ES ejection sound
electrical stimulation
emergency services
exterior surface

ESA end-to-side anastomosis
evidence of sexual abuse

ESB electrical stimulation of the brain

ESC end-systolic counts (cardiology)
enhanced serum cortisol

ESD esophagus, stomach, duodenum

ESE	endoscopic excision
ESEG	echosonoencephalogram
ESF	erythropoietic stimulating factor
ESG	electrospinogram
ESGD	end-to-side gastroduodenostomy
ESHD	end-stage heart disease
ESKD	end-stage kidney disease
ESLD	end-stage liver disease
ESM	ejection systolic murmur
ESO	electrically stimulated osteogenesis esophagus
ESP	end-systolic pressure extrasensory perception
ESR	electric skin response erythrocyte sedimentation rate (laboratory/hematology)
ESRD	end-stage renal disease
ESS	empty sella syndrome erythrocyte sensitizing substance expiratory standstill (pulmonary medicine)
ess	essential
EST	electroshock therapy (procedure/psychiatry)
est	estimated

esu	electrostatic unit
ESV	end-systolic volume
ET	ejection time endotracheal tube esotropia (eye examination) eustachian tube
ETA	endotracheal aspirates
et al	and others (Latin: *et alii*)
ETAP	epidemic tropical acute polyarthritis
ETD	estimated time of death
ETH/C	elixir terpin hydrate with codeine (medication order)
ETI	ejection time index endotracheal intubation
etiol	etiology
ETK	every test known
ETM	erythromycin (on culture and sensitivity reports)
ETO	estimated time of ovulation
ETOH	ethyl alcohol
ETP	elective termination of pregnancy entire treatment period
ETR	effective thyroxine ratio (nuclear medicine)
ETT	endotracheal tube

ETT *(cont)*	exercise tolerance test eye tracking test
ETU	emergency treatment unit
EU	emergency unit enzyme units
EUA	examination under anesthetic (procedure/gynecology)
EUCD	emotionally unstable character disorder
EUG	echouterogram
EUL	expected upper limit
EV	extravascular
ev	electron-volt
evac	evacuate
eval	evaluate
EVR	evoked visual response
EW	emergency ward
EWB	estrogen withdrawal bleeding
EWL	evaporative water loss
EX	excision
ex	examined example
EXBF	exercise hyperemia blood flow

exc	except excision
ExD	exertional dyspnea
ExFHR	external fetal heart rate (monitoring)
EXO	extraction (dentistry)
exp	expected expectorated expired exploration
expir	expiration
exp lap	exploratory laparotomy (operation/abdominal)
expt	expectorant
ExREM	external radiation dose
ext	extension extensor external extract extremity
ExU	excretory urogram
exx	examples
Ez	eczema

F

F	factor Fahrenheit false family farad father feces female fetal filament function
f	fluid focal frequency from
F_1, F_2	filial generations (first, second)
FA	false aneurysm fatty acid femoral artery fetal age field ambulance filtered air first aid folic acid forearm
F/A	fetus active financial arrangements
FAB	functional arm brace
FABER	flexion in abduction and external rotation
FAC	fluorouracil, adriamycin, cyclophosphamide (chemotherapy)

FAD	familial Alzheimer's disease
FAI	first aid instruction functional aerobic impairment
FAM	fibroadenomyxoma
FANA	fluorescent antinuclear antibodies (laboratory/chemistry
FAP	familial adenomatous polyposis familial amyloid polyneuropathy
FAS	fetal alcohol syndrome fluorescent antibody staining
FAST	fluorescent allergosorbent test (allergy)
FAT	feminizing adrenal tumor fluorescent antibody test food awareness training
FAVA	facioauriculovertebral anomaly
FB	feedback finger breadth foreign body
FBC	full blood count
FBD	functional bowel disorder
FBG	fasting blood glucose
FBI	flossing, brushing, irrigation (dentistry)
FBP	familial benign pemphigus femoral blood pressure
FBS	fasting blood sugar (laboratory/chemistry)

FBT	family-based treatment
FBW	fasting blood work
FC	family conference finger-counting (eye examination) Foley catheter
F/C	fever and chills
F & C	foam and condom (gynecology)
FCC	fracture, compound and comminuted
FCD	familial corneal dystrophy fibrocystic disease (mammography finding)
FCG	French catheter gauge
FCH	familial clitoral hypertrophy
FCMC	family-centered maternity care
FCR	Fuji computed radiography
FCS	facial cosmetic surgery familial centrolobar sclerosis
FCT	food control training
FD	fatal dose focal distance (eye examination) foot drape forceps delivery
F/D	fracture dislocation
F & D	fixed and dilated (ophthalmology)
Fd	fundus

FDA	Food and Drug Administration
FDC	follicular dendritic cell
FDDS	former dentist
fdg	feeding
FDH	focal dermal hypoplasia
FDIU	fetal death in utero
FDP	fibrin degradation product (laboratory/coagulation)
FDS	fetal distress syndrome (fetal asphyxia) for duration of stay (hospital)
FE	fat embolism female escutcheon fibroepithelioma fluid extract
Fe	iron (Latin: *ferrum*)
^{59}Fe	radioactive iron (nuclear medicine)
FEA	familial erythroblastic anemia
feb agg	febrile agglutinin (laboratory/serology)
FEC	familial erythrocytosis
FECG	fetal electrocardiogram (procedure/obstetrics)
FECT	fibroelastic connective tissue
FECV	functional extracellular fluid volume

Fe def	iron deficiency (anemia)
FEEG	fetal electroencephalogram
FEF	forced expiratory flow (pulmonary function test)
FELV	feline leukemia virus
fem	female (feminine) femoral
FEN	fluid, electrolytes, nutrition
FES	fat embolism syndrome flame emission spectroscopy forced expiratory spirogram (pulmonary function test) functional electrical stimulation
FESS	functional endoscopic sinus surgery
FET	forced expiratory time (pulmonary function test)
FETI	fluorescence energy transfer immunoassay
FETS	forced expiratory time in seconds (pulmonary function test)
FEUO	for external use only (medications)
FEV	forced expiratory volume (pulmonary function test)
FEV_1	forced expiratory volume in one second (pulmonary function test)
FF	factitious fever

FF *(cont)*	fat-free (diet) finger to finger (neurological examination) flat feet force fluids (diet order) foster father fresh frozen
f/f	fundus firm (obstetrics)
FFA	free fatty acids (laboratory/chemistry) fluorescein fundus angiogram (procedure/ophthalmology)
FFB	flexible fiberoptic bronchoscope
FFC	fixed flexion contracture (orthopedics)
FFD	focus-to-film distance (x-ray)
FFDW	fat-free dry weight
FFI	free from infection
FFM	fat-free mass
FFP	familial periodic paralysis fresh frozen plasma
FFQ	fecal fat quantitation
FFS	fee for service flexible fiberoptic sigmoidoscopy
FGC	full gold crown (dentistry)
FGT	female genital tract
FH	family history fetal head fetal heart

FHA familial hemolytic anemia

FHC family health center

FHI familial hemolytic icterus

FHIP family health insurance plan

FHMI family history of mental illness

FHN familial hemorrhagic nephritis
femoral head necrosis

FHNH fetal heart not heard

FHO family history of obesity

FHPD familial hyperplastic periosteal dystrophy

FHR fetal heart rate

FHS fetal heart sounds
functional hiatal stenosis

FHx family history

FI focal infection
food intake
forced inspiration
functionally impaired

FIA fluorescence immunoassay

fib fibrillation

fibrin fibrinogen (laboratory/coagulation)

$FICO_2$ concentration of carbon dioxide in inspired gas (respiratory therapy)

FICU	fetal intensive care unit
FIF	forced inspiratory flow (pulmonary function test)
fig	figure
FIH	fat-induced hyperglycemia
FIHJ	familial intrahepatic jaundice
FIHL	fat-induced hyperlipemia
FIN	fine intestinal needle
FIO_2	concentration of oxygen in inspired gas (respiratory therapy)
FIP	fibrosing interstitial pneumonitis
FISH	fluorescence in situ hybridization
fist	fistula
FIT	food intolerance testing
FIUO	for internal use only (medications)
FIVC	forced inspiratory vital capacity
FJN	familial juvenile nephrophthisis
FJRM	full joint range of motion
FL	focal length frontal lobe
fl	fluid flutter

FLB funny looking beat (ECG)

fld field

fl dr fluid dram

fl ext fluid extract

fl oz fluid ounce

FLSA follicular lymphosarcoma

Fl tx fluoride treatment (dentistry)

fluor fluorescent
fluoroscopy (procedure/radiology)

fl up flare up
follow up

FM face mask
fetal movements
flowmeter
foreign matter
forensic medicine

F & M firm and midline (uterus)

FMA familial microcytic anemia

FMC fetal movement count

FMD familial metaphyseal dysplasia
fibromuscular dysplasia
foot and mouth disease (infectious diseases)
former medical doctor

FME full mouth extraction (operation/oral surgery)

FMF	familial Mediterranean fever forced midexpiratory flow
FMG	fine mesh gauze foreign medical graduate
FMH	fetal-maternal hemorrhage
FMP	first menstrual period
FMS	false memory syndrome fat-mobilizing substances full mouth series (dentistry)
FMT	functional maintenance therapy (geriatrics)
FMX	full mouth x-rays (dentistry)
FN	false-negative finger to nose (neurological examination)
FNA	fine needle aspiration (biopsy)
FNB	flat nasal bridge
FNH	focal nodular hyperplasia
FNHJ	familial nonhemolytic jaundice
FNL	familial neurovisceral lipidosis
FNP	Family Nurse Practitioner
FNS	functional neuromuscular stimulation
FO	familial occurrence foramen ovale (heart) foreign object frontooccipital

FOB	fiberoptic bronchoscopy foot of bed
FOBT	fecal occult blood test
FOC	father of child
FOCS	familial ovarian cancer syndromes
FOD	familial osseous dystrophy free of disease
FOE	fiberoptic examination
Fol cath	Foley catheter
FOO	foreign object obstruction
FOOB	fell out of bed
FOP	fiberoptic probe
FOVI	field of vision intact (ophthalmology)
FOW	fenestrated oval window (operation/otology)
FP	facial palsy false-positive family planning family practice flat plate (x-ray/abdomen) fluid pressure frozen plasma
FPB	femoropopliteal bypass (cardiology)
FPC	familial paroxysmal choreoathetosis family practice center frozen packed cells

FPD	fetopelvic disproportion (obstetrics) fixed partial denture
FPG	fasting plasma glucose
FPHx	family psychiatric history
FPIA	fluorescence polarization immunoassay
FPNA	first-pass nuclear angiocardiography
FPS	facial plastic surgery
FR	failure rate flow rate fluid retention
Fr	French (catheter gauge)
F & R	force and rhythm (of pulse)
FRA	fluorescent rabies antibody (test)
FRC	frozen red cells functional reserve capacity (of lungs) (pulmonary function test) functional residual capacity (of lungs) (pulmonary function test)
freq	frequent
FRF	follicle-stimulating hormone releasing factor (laboratory/endocrinology)
frict	friction (rub)
FRJM	full-range joint movement
FROM	full range of motion

FRP	familial recurring polyserositis functional refractory period (neurology)
FRS	facial reconstructive surgery
FRT	full recovery time
FRV	functional residual volume
FS	fracture, simple frozen section full and soft (diet order) function study
FSA	familial splenic anemia
FSB	fetal scalp blood (fetal monitoring)
FSBM	full-strength breast milk
FSC	fracture, simple, comminuted
FSD	focus-to-skin distance (x-ray)
FSE	fetal scalp electrode
FSF	fibrin stabilizing factor (Factor XIII) (laboratory/coagulation)
FSH	follicle-stimulating hormone (laboratory/endocrinology)
FSI	fasting serum insulin
FSMD	facioscapulohumeral muscular dystrophy
FSP	familial spastic paraplegia fibrin split products

FSPG	focal segmental proliferative glomerulonephritis
FT	family therapy feeding tube fibrous tissue follow through (after barium meal) (x-ray/intestines) full-term (obstetrics)
FT_3	free triiodothyronine (laboratory/endocrinology)
FT_4	free thyroxine (laboratory/endocrinology)
FTA	fluorescent treponemal antibodies (syphilis) (laboratory/serology)
FTA-Abs	fluorescent treponemal antibody absorption (test) (laboratory/serology)
FTAG	fast-binding, target-attaching globulin
FTBD	full-term, born dead
FTD	failure to descend (obstetrics)
FTE	free thyroxine equivalent (laboratory/endocrinology)
FTF	free thyroxine fraction
FTG	full-thickness graft (operation/plastic surgery)
FTI	free thyroxine index (laboratory/endocrinology)
FTM	fractional test meal

FTND	full-term normal delivery
FTP	failure to progress (in labor) (obstetrics)
FTR	for the record
FTSG	full-thickness skin graft
FTT	failure to thrive (pediatrics)
FU	fat unit fecal urobilinogen (laboratory/chemistry)
5-FU	5-fluorouracil (chemotherapy)
f/u	follow up
FUB	functional uterine bleeding
FUN	follow-up note (medical records)
FUO	fever of unknown origin
FUT	fibrinogen uptake test
FUV	follow-up visit
FV	femoral vein fluid volume
FVA	four-vessel arteriography (cardiology)
FVC	forced vital capacity (pulmonary function test)
FVE	forced volume, expiratory (pulmonary function test)
FVH	focal vascular headache

FVL	femoral vein ligation
FVU	first voided urine
FW	fragment wound
FWB	full weight bearing
FWOC	fine without changing
FWR	Felix-Weil reaction (laboratory/serology)
FWW	front-wheel walker
Fx	fracture
Fx BB	fracture of both bones
Fx Dis	fracture-dislocation
FXN	function
FXS	fragile X syndrome
fxur	fractional urine
FZ	focal zone frozen section

G

G	gallop (cardiology) gas globulin glucose good grade gravid green guanine guttae
g	acceleration due to gravity gram group
GA	gastric analysis general anesthesia general appearance gestational age
^{67}Ga	radioactive gallium (nuclear medicine)
ga	gauge (of needles)
g/a	ginger ale (diet order)
GAD	generalized anxiety disorder
GADS	gonococcal arthritis/dermatitis syndrome
GAF	global assessment of functioning
gal	gallon
GALT	gut-associated lymphoid tissue
garg	gargle

GAS	gastroenterology
GaS	gallium scan
GASA	glove-and-stocking anesthesia
GASTS	group A streptococcal toxic shock
GAT	glutamic acid toxicity (Chinese restaurant syndrome)
GB	gallbladder
GBA	ganglionic blocking agent
GBBS	group B beta-hemolytic streptococcus
GBM	glomerular basement membrane
GBS	gallbladder series gastric bypass surgery Guillain-Barré syndrome
GC	gas chromatography gonococcus (gonorrhea) geriatric care granular casts (urine)
GCA	giant-cell arteritis
g-cal	gram-calorie
GCC	granular cell carcinoma
GCD	granular corneal dystrophy
GCFT	gonorrhea complement fixation test
GCL	giant-cell leukemia

g-cm	gram-centimeter
GCMB	granular cell myoblastoma
GCMS	granular cell myosarcoma
GCNF	granular cell neurofibroma
GCS	giant-cell sarcoma
GCSE	generalized convulsive status epilepticus
GCT	giant-cell tumor granular cell tumor
GCX	giant-cell xanthoma
GD	given dose gonadal dysgenesis (urology) Graves' disease
G & D	growth & development (pediatrics)
gd	good
GDH	gonadotropic hormone
GDM	gestational diabetes mellitus
GDS	Geriatric Depression Scale gradual dosage scale
GDT	goal-directed therapy
GE	gastroenterology gastroenterostomy (operation/stomach) gastroesophageal
G/E	granulocyte-erythroid ratio (laboratory/hematology)

GEA general anesthesia

GEF gonadotropin enhancing factor

GEJ gastroesophageal junction

gen general

gent genital
gentamicin

GEP gel electrophoresis

GER gastroesophageal reflux
geriatrics

GERD gastroesophageal reflux disorder

GES glucose electrolyte solution

GET gastric emptying time

GF girlfriend
glomerular filtration
gluten-free (diet order)
grandfather
growth fraction

GFAP glial fibrillary acidic protein

GFD gluten-free diet (diet order)

GFL giant follicular lymphoma

GFLB giant follicular lymphoblastoma

GFM gingival fibromatosis

GFR glomerular filtration rate

GG	galloping gangrene (necrotizing fasciitis) gammaglobulin
GGE	generalized glandular enlargement
GGS	glands, goiter, stiffness (neck examination)
GGT	gamma glutamyl transferase (laboratory/liver function)
GH	general hospital growth hormone (laboratory/endocrinology)
GHD	growth hormone deficiency
GHF	growth hormone failure
GHQ	general health questionnaire
GHRF	growth hormone releasing factor (laboratory/endocrinology)
GI	gastrointestinal gelatin infusion gender identity globin insulin guided imagery (psychiatry)
GIA	gastrointestinal anastomosis
GIB	gastric ileal bypass
GIBF	gastrointestinal bacterial flora
GIFAM	giant intracanalicular fibroadenomyxoma
GIFT	gamete intrafallopian transfer (artificial insemination)
GIH	growth-inhibiting hormone

GIK	glucose, insulin and potassium (intravenous solution)
GIP	gastric inhibitory polypeptide gastrointestinal polyposis
GIPU	gastrointestinal postburn ulcer
GIS	gas in stomach gastrointestinal series (x-ray/stomach) gastrointestinal system
GIT	gastrointestinal tract glucose infusion test (diabetes detection)
GITT	glucose-insulin tolerance test
GIV	gastrointestinal virus
GJ	gastrojejunostomy
GJLO	gastrojejunal loop obstruction
GL	glaucoma
gl	gland
GLC	gas-liquid chromatography
GLD	globoid leukodystrophy
GLH	glossolabial hemispasm
GLL	glycolipid lipidosis
Gln	glutamine
glob	globulin (laboratory/chemistry)
GLP	group living program

GLPP glossolabiopharyngeal paralysis

Glu glutamate

gluc glucose

GM gastric mucosa
gentamicin (on culture and sensitivity reports)
grand mal (seizure)
grandmother
grand multiparity

Gm gram

Gm- Gram stain negative (on bacteriology reports)

Gm+ Gram stain positive (on bacteriology reports)

GM % grams per hundred milliliters

GMA goat's milk anemia

GMAT general medical action team (emergency medicine)

GMC globulomaxillary cyst

GM-CSF granulocyte-macrophage colony-stimulating factor

GMM giant mammary myxoma

gm-m gram-meter

GMS grand mal seizure
General Medical Services

GMW gram molecular weight

GN glomerulonephritis
graduate nurse
gram-negative

G/N glucose-nitrogen (ratio)

Gn gonadotropin

GNB gram-negative bacilli

GNC gram-negative cocci

GNID gram-negative intracellular diplococci

GnRH gonadotropin-releasing hormone

G/NS glucose in normal saline
(intravenous solution)

GO glucose oxidase
gynecooncology
generalized obesity

GOE gas, oxygen, ether (anesthesia)

GOO gastric outlet obstruction

GP general paralysis
general paresis
general practitioner
gram-positive

GPB glossopharyngeal breathing

GPC gram-positive cocci

G6PD glucose-6-phosphate dehydrogenase
(laboratory/chemistry)

GPH gonococcal perihepatitis

GPKA guinea pig kidney absorption test (laboratory/serology)

GPLP glossopalatolabial paralysis

GPM general preventive medicine

GPP glossopharyngeal paralysis

GpTh group therapy (psychiatry)

GR gastric resection (operation/stomach)

gr grain (medication orders/prescriptions)
gravity

GRA gonadotropin-releasing agent

grad gradient
gradually
graduated

GRAE generally recognized as effective

gran granular

GRAS generally recognized as safe

grav gravida (pregnancy)
gravity

grav ī primigravida (first pregnancy)

grav ī/Ab ī one pregnancy, one abortion

grav ō no pregnancies

GRBAS grade, rough, breathy, asthenic, strained

GRD	gastroesophageal reflux disease
GRE	graduated resistance exercise (physical therapy)
GRF	gonadotropin-releasing factor (laboratory/endocrinology)
GRH	growth hormone-releasing hormone
GRIF	growth hormone release-inhibiting factor
GRT	good response to treatment
GS	gallstone general surgery glomerular sclerosis gut sutures
G/S	glucose and saline (intravenous solution)
GSC	gas-solid chromatography
GSD	glycogen storage disease
GSE	gluten-sensitive enteropathy grips strong and equal (physical therapy)
GSH	growth-stimulating hormone
GSR	galvanic skin response
GSV	great saphenous vein
GSW	gunshot wound
GT	gait training (physical therapy) gastrostomy tube genetic therapy glucose tolerance

GT *(cont)*	glutamyl transferase (liver function test)
GTA	global transient amnesia
GTF	glucose tolerance factor
GTH	gonadotropic hormone (laboratory/endocrinology)
GTI	genital tract infection
GTN	glyceryl trinitrate (nitroglycerine)
GTT	glucose tolerance test (diabetes detection)
gtts	drops (Latin: *guttae*) (medication orders/prescriptions)
GU	gastric ulcer genitourinary gonococcal urethritis
GUD	genital ulcer disease
GUS	genitourinary system
GV	gentian violet (dye) gingivectomy (dentistry)
GVHD	graft versus host disease
GVHR	graft versus host reaction
GW	gunshot wound
G/W	glucose in water (intravenous solution)
GWE	glycerin and water enema
GWS	Gulf War syndrome (toxicology)

GXT	graded exercise test (procedure/cardiology)
GYN	gynecology
GZI	globin zinc insulin

H

H	head heart hernia heroin horizontal hormone hospital human husband hydrogen hypermetropia (eye examination)
(H)	hypodermic injection (medication order)
H_1, H_2	histamine receptor (type 1, type 2)
H+	hydrogen ion
h	height hour
h^2	heritability (genetics)
HA	headache hearing aid heated aerosol hemadsorbent hemagglutination hemolytic anemia hepatic adenoma hepatitis A heterophil antibody (infectious mononucleosis) hospital admission
H/A	height/age
Ha	absolute hypermetropia (eye examination)

HA1, HA2	hemadsorption virus (type 1, type 2)
HAA	hearing aid amplifier hemolytic anemia antigen hepatitis-associated antigen (Australian antigen)
HAAb	hepatitis A antibody
HAAg	hepatitis A antigen
HAAS	Havighurst Activities and Attitudes Scale
HAb	heart antibody
HAD	hospital administration
HAE	hearing aid evaluation hereditary angioneurotic edema
HAG	height-age-gender
HAGG	hyperimmune antivariola gammaglobulin
HAI	hemagglutination inhibition hepatic arterial infusion hospital-acquired infection
HAL	hyperalimentation
HAN	heroin-associated nephropathy
HAP	home antibiotic program
HAPE	high-altitude pulmonary edema
HAPS	hepatic arterial perfusion scintigraphy
HAS	hypertensive arteriosclerosis

HASCVD hypertensive arteriosclerotic cardiovascular disease

HASHD hypertensive arteriosclerotic heart disease

HAT head, arms, trunk
hospital arrival time
hyperazotemia

HATT hemagglutination treponemal test

HAV hepatitis A virus

HB His bundle
hold breakfast
hospital-based
hospital bed

HB1°-3° heart block (first, second and third degree)

Hb (Hgb) hemoglobin

HbA normal adult hemoglobin

HBAb hepatitis B antibody

HBAg hepatitis B antigen

HbAS hemoglobin A and hemoglobin S (sickle cell trait)

HBB hospital blood bank

HB/BW hold breakfast for blood work

HBD alpha-hydroxybutyric dehydrogenase
has been drinking

HBDH hydroxybutyric dehydrogenase

HBE	His bundle electrogram
HBeAg	hepatitis B e antigen
HBF	hepatic blood flow
Hb-F	fetal hemoglobin
HBGM	home blood glucose monitoring
HBI	hepatobiliary imaging
HBIG	hepatitis B immunoglobulin
HBO	hyperbaric oxygen
H_3BO_3	boric acid
HbO_2	oxyhemoglobin
HBP	high blood pressure hospital-based physician hysterical back pain
HBS	hyperkinetic behavior syndrome
HbS	sickle cell hemoglobin
HBsAb	hepatitis B surface antibody
HBsAg	hepatitis B surface antigen
HBT	hereditary benign tremor
HBV	hepatitis B vaccine hepatitis B virus
HBW	high birth weight

HC handicapped
head compression
health care
hepatic coma
home care
house call
Huntington's chorea (neurology)
hyaline casts (urine)
hydrocortisone

HCA health care aide
hydrocortisone acetate
hypochromic anemia
hypoplastic congenital anemia

HCC hepatocellular carcinoma
history of chief complaint
hydroxycholecalciferol (Vitamin D)

HCD health care delivery
heavy chain disease
hysterical conversion disorder

HCE human chorionic erlichiosis
(pseudo-Lyme disease)

HCF hereditary capillary fragility
high carbohydrate foods

HCG human chorionic gonadotropin
(laboratory/endocrinology)

HChA hypochromic anemia

HCHF high carbohydrate, high fiber (diet)

HCHO formaldehyde

HCL hairy cell leukemia
hard contact lens

HCl	hydrochloric acid hydrochloride
HCLF	high carbohydrate, low fiber (diet)
HCM	health care maintenance hyperchylomicronemia hypertrophic cardiomyopathy
HCO_3	bicarbonate
HCP	health care plan hexachlorophene
HCPP	health care payment plan
HCR	hysterical conversion reaction (psychiatry)
HCSM	human chorionic somatomammotropin
HCT	histamine challenge test human calcitonin human chorionic thyrotropin
Hct (also hct)	hematocrit (laboratory/hematology)
HCTU	home cervical traction unit (physical therapy)
HCTZ	hydrochlorothiazide
HCU	heterochromic uveitis homocystinuria
HCV	hepatitis C virus
HCVD	hypertensive cardiovascular disease
HCW	health care worker

HD	hearing distance heart disease hemodialysis herniated disc high-density Hodgkin's disease hospital day
HDA	histiocytic dermoarthritis
HDBH	hydroxybutyric dehydrogenase
HDC	human diploid cell
HDF	hereditary dysfibrinoginemia host defensive factor
HDH	heart disease history
HDL	high-density lipoproteins
HDN	hemolytic disease of the newborn high-density nebulizer
HDNS	hereditary dysplastic nevus syndrome (dermatology)
HDR	hysterical dissociative reaction (psychiatry)
HDS	health delivery system herniated disc syndrome
HDU	hemodialysis unit
HDV	hepatitis D (delta) virus
HDW	hearing distance with watch

HE	hard exudate (ophthalmology) hemoglobin electrophoresis
H & E	hematoxylin and eosin (stain) hemorrhage and exudate heredity and environment
HEA	hereditary elliptocytic anemia
HEAT	human erythrocyte agglutination test
HEC	health education center hospital ethics committee
HED	hidrotic ectodermal dysplasia
HEENT	head, ears, eyes, nose, throat
HEG	hemorrhagic erosive gastritis
HEK	human embryonic kidney
HEL	human embryonic lung
HELLP	hemolysis, elevated liver enzymes, low platelets (syndrome)
HEMPAS	hereditary erythroblastic multinuclearity with positive acidified serum
HEN	hemorrhage, exudates, nicking (ophthalmology)
HEPA	high-efficiency particulate air
HES	hypereosinophilic syndrome
HEV	hepatitis E virus human enteric virus

HF	Hageman factor (laboratory/coagulation) hard fibroma harlequin fetus hay fever heart failure hemorrhagic fever high fat high frequency Hispanic female
HFA	health facility administrator hyperfolic acidemia
HFAK	hollow-fiber artificial kidney
HFC	hard-filled capsules
HFD	high forceps delivery
HFHL	high-frequency hearing loss
HFI	hereditary fructose intolerance high fat intake
HFJV	high-frequency jet ventilation
HFOV	high-frequency oscillatory ventilation
HFPPV	high-frequency positive pressure ventilation
HFRS	hemorrhagic fever with renal syndrome
HFUPR	hourly fetal urine production rate
HFV	high-frequency ventilation
HG	herpes genitalis human gonadotropin

Hg	mercury (Latin: *hydrargyrum*)
HGF	human growth factor hyperglycemic factor
Hg-F	fetal hemoglobin
HGG	human gammaglobulin
HGH	human growth hormone
HGO	hepatic glucose output
HH	hard of hearing hiatal hernia home hyperalimentation
H & H	hemoglobin and hematocrit
HHA	hereditary hemolytic anemia home health aide
HHb	reduced hemoglobin
HHC	home health care
HHD	hypertensive heart disease
HHE	hemiconvulsions, hemiplegia, epilepsy (syndrome)
HHG	hypogonadotropic hypogonadism
HHHO	hypotonia, hypomentia, hypogonadism, obesity
HHM	high-humidity mask
HHN	hand-held nebulizer home health nurse

HHNC	hyperglycemic hyperosmolar nonketotic coma
HHO	home health organization
HHS	history of heavy smoking
HHT	hereditary hemorrhagic telangiectasia
HHV	human herpesvirus
HI	head injury health insurance hemagglutination inhibition hepatic insufficiency hepatobiliary imaging
Hi	histidine
HIA	hemagglutination inhibition antibody
5-HIAA	5-hydroxyindoleacetic acid
HIB	Haemophyllus influenzae (type B)
HIC	heart information center
HID	headache, insomnia, depression hyperkinetic impulse disorder
HIF	higher integrative functions (neurology)
HIH	Halsted's inguinal herniorrhaphy
HIHA	high impulsiveness, high anxiety
HII	hemagglutination-inhibition immunoassay
HIIN	hypertrophic interstitial infantile neuritis

HILA	high impulsiveness, low anxiety
HIN	health insurance network
H & IO	hernia and intestinal obstruction
HIP	hospital insurance program
Hip B	Hippocratic baldness (dermatology)
HIRO	hormonal imbalance related to ovulation
HIS	health information service high index of suspicion human immune system
Hist X	histiocytosis X
HIT	hemagglutination-inhibition test
HIV	human immunodeficiency virus (AIDS)
HIVD	herniated intervertebral disc
HJB	Howell-Jolly bodies
HJR	hepatojugular reflex
H-K	hand to knee heat-killed heel to knee
HKA	hypokalemic alkalosis
HKC	human kidney cells
HKO	hip-knee orthosis (splint)
HL	hair line

HL *(cont)*	half-life (of a radioactive element) harelip hearing loss Hodgkin's lymphoma hyperlipidemia
H & L	heart and lungs
Hl	hypermetropia, latent (eye examination)
HLA	human leukocyte antigen human lymphocyte antibody
HLD	herniated lumbar disc
HLH	human luteinizing hormone
HLI	hemolysis inhibition
HLK	heart, liver, kidneys
HLP	hyperlipoproteinemia
HLR	heart-lung resuscitation
HLTK	Holmium laser thermokeratoplasty
HLV	herpes-like virus
HM	hand movements heart murmur Hispanic male hydatidiform mole
Hm	hypermetropia, manifest (eye examination)
HMC	heroin, morphine, cocaine
HMD	hyaline membrane disease

HME	heat, massage, exercise (physical therapy)
HMG	human menopausal gonadotropin
HMI	healed myocardial infarction history of medical illness
HM & LP	hand motion and light perception (neurology)
HMM	home maintenance management (nursing)
HMO	Health Maintenance Organization heart minute output
HMP	hot moist packs (physical therapy)
HMW	high-molecular-weight
HN	Head Nurse high nitrogen
HN_2	nitrogen mustard (medication order)
H & N	head and neck
HNA	headache, nausea, anorexia hereditary neuropathic amyloidosis
HNCD	hereditary nonprogressive corneal dystrophy
HNO_3	nitric acid
HNP	herniated nucleus pulposus
hnRNA	heterogeneous nuclear ribonucleic acid
HNS	head and neck surgery

HNSHA	hereditary nonspherocytic hemolytic anemia
HNV	has not voided
HnV	hantavirus
HO	House Officer (intern or resident physician) hyperbaric oxygen
h/o	history of
H_2O	water
H_2O_2	hydrogen peroxide
HOB	head of bed
HOBC	hereditary ovarian/breast cancer
HOC	hereditary ovalocytosis human ovarian cancer
HOCM	hypertrophic obstructive cardiomyopathy
HOD	hyperbaric oxygen drenching (sports medicine)
HOF	height of fundus
HOH	hard of hearing
HOM	habronemic ophthalmomyiasis
HOP	high oxygen pressure (respiratory therapy)
HOPA	hospital-based organ procurement agency
HOPD	hospital outpatient department

HOS	human osteosarcoma
HP	handicapped person hard palate health plan health professional hemiplegia high potency high power high protein (diet order) hot pack (pad) House Physician hydrostatic pressure
Hp	haptoglobin
H & P	history and physical (examination)
HPA	hypothalamic-pituitary-adrenal (axis)
HPD	high-protein diet
HPE	history and physical examination
hpf	high-power field (microscopy)
HPFH	hereditary persistence of fetal hemoglobin
HPG	human pituitary gonadotropin hypothalamic-pituitary-gonadal (axis)
HPHO	hyperplastic hyperostosis
HPI	history of present illness
HPL	human placental lactogen
HPLC	high-pressure liquid chromatography
HPM	hemiplegic migraine

HPN	home parenteral nutrition
HPO	high-pressure oxygen (respiratory therapy) hypothalamic-pituitary-ovarian (axis)
HPP	hyperplastic periostosis
HPR	hospital peer review
HPr	human prolactin
HPS	hantavirus pulmonary syndrome high-protein supplement hypertrophic pyloric stenosis
HPT	human placenta thyrotropin hyperparathyroidism hypothalamic-pituitary-testicular (axis)
HPTh	hypothalamic-pituitary-thyroidal (axis)
HPV	human papillomavirus
HPVD	hypertensive pulmonary vascular disease
HPZ	high pressure zone
HR	heart rate hospital record
hr	hour
H & R	hysterectomy and radiation
HRA	heart rate audiometry high right atrial (ECG)
HRCT	high resolution computer tomography
HRF	histamine releasing factor

HRG	health research group
HRIG	human rabies immune globulin (medication order)
HRL	head rotated left
HRM	Halsted's radical mastectomy
HRR	head retraction reflex head rotated right
HRS	hepatorenal syndrome
HRT	hormone replacement therapy
HRtV	human rotavirus
HRVLA	human reovirus-like agent
HS	half strength hand surgery Hartman's solution (intravenous solution) heart sounds heat stable heel spur hereditary spherocytosis herpes simplex horse serum House Surgeon Hurler's syndrome
hs	at bedtime (Latin: *hora somni*) (medication orders/prescriptions) hour of sleep
HSA	health services agreement human serum albumin (medication order) hypersomnia-sleep apnea

HSAN	head shaking after nystagmus
HSAS	hypertrophic subaortic stenosis
HSCD	Hand-Schüller-Christian disease
HSDI	Health Self-Determination Index
HSE	herpes simplex encephalitis
HSG	hysterosalpingogram
hSGF	human skeletal growth factor
HSM	hepatosplenomegaly holosystolic murmur (cardiology)
H_2SO_4	sulfuric acid
HSP	health systems plan Henoch-Schönlein purpura
HSQ	home screening questionnaire
HSRD	hypertension secondary to renal disease
HST	health screening test
HSTS	human-specific thyroid stimulator
HSV	herpes simplex virus
HT	hammer toe head trauma hearing test high temperature home treatment hydrotherapy (physical therapy) hypnotherapy

HT *(cont)*	hypodermic tablet hypothalamus
5-HT	5-hydroxytryptamine (serotonin)
Ht	hypermetropia, total (eye examination)
HTAT	human tetanus antitoxin
HTB	hot tub bath (physical therapy)
HTE	hypertensive encephalopathy
HTLV	human T-cell lymphotropic virus (AIDS retrovirus)
HTN	hypertension
HTS	hemangioma-thrombocytopenia syndrome human thyroid stimulator
HTV	herpes-type virus
HU	heat unit hydroxyurea hyperemia unit
HUAM	home uterine activity monitoring
HuIF	human interferon
HUIS	high-dose urea in invert sugar
HUM	heat, ultrasound, massage
HURT	hospital utilization review team
HUS	hemolytic uremic syndrome

HV	has voided hepatic vein herpesvirus hospital visit hyperventilation
H & V	hemigastrectomy and vagotomy
HVA	homovanillic acid (assay) (laboratory/endocrinology)
HVD	hypertensive vascular disease
HVE	hepatic vascular exclusion high-voltage electrophoresis
HVG	host versus graft (response)
HVH	herpesvirus hominis
HVL	half-value layer (radiology)
HVR	hypoxic ventilatory response (pulmonary medicine)
HVT	half-value thickness (radiology) hepatic vein thrombosis
HWB	hot water bottle
HWS	hot water soluble
Hx	history hospitalization
Hy	hypermetropia (eye examination)
hyd	hydration
hydro	hydrotherapy (physical therapy)

hyg	hygiene
HYP	hypnosis (psychiatry)
hyp	hypertrophy
hypo	hypodermic injection
hys	hysteria
hyst	hysterectomy
HZ	herpes zoster (virus)
Hz	Hertz (electrical measurement)

I

I
inactive
incisor
index
induction (anesthesia)
inhibitor
intake
iodine

^{125}I, ^{131}I
radioactive iodine (nuclear medicine)

i
increased
insoluble

IA
image amplification (radiology)
imperforate anus
incidental appendectomy (operation/abdominal)
infected area
internal auditory (ear)
intraarterial (blood pressure)
intraarticular (injection)

I & A
irrigation and aspiration (ophthalmology)

IABC
intraaortic balloon counterpulsation (procedure/cardiology)

IABP
intraaortic balloon pump

IAC
internal auditory canal
interposed abdominal compression
intraarticular calcification

IACP
intraaortic counterpulsation

IAD
internal absorbed dose (radiology)

IADHS	inappropriate antidiuretic hormone syndrome
IADL	Instrumental Activities of Daily Living (scale)
IAE	intraatrial electrocardiogram
IAH	implantable artificial heart
IAHA	immune adherence hemagglutination
IAI	intraabdominal infection
IAM	internal auditory meatus
IAO	immediately after onset
IAP	immunosuppressive acidic protein
IAPT	idiopathic auricular paroxysmal tachycardia
IAS	intraamniotic saline (infusion) (procedure/gynecology)
IASD	intraatrial septal defect (heart)
IAT	indirect antiglobulin test
IAV	intermittent assisted ventilation
IB	inclusion body infectious bronchitis isolation bed
IBC	intraaortic balloon counterpulsation (cardiology) iron-binding capacity (laboratory/chemistry)

IBD	inflammatory bowel disease
IBE	inclusion body encephalitis
IBF	immunoglobulin-binding factor intermittent biliary fever
IBI	intermittent bladder irrigation (procedure/urology)
IBL	immunoblastic lymphadenopathy
IBNR	incurred but not reported
IBP	iron-binding protein
IBPMS	indirect blood pressure measuring system
IBS	irritable bowel syndrome
IBT	inkblot (Rorschach) test
IBV	infectious bronchitis virus
IBW	ideal body weight
IC	immune complex indirect calorimetry individual counseling (psychiatry) infection control inspiratory capacity (pulmonary function test) intensive care intercostal intermediate care interstitial cells intracapsular intracavitary intracellular intracerebral

IC *(cont)*	intracranial intracutaneous (injection site) irritable colon isovolumic contraction (heart)
I/C	incomplete
I & C	incision and curettage
ICA	internal carotid artery intracranial aneurysm
ICAM	intercellular adhesion molecule
ICBP	intracellular binding protein
ICC	intensive coronary care
ICCE	intracapsular cataract extraction (operation/ophthalmology)
ICCEPI	intracapsular cataract extraction with peripheral iridectomy (operation/ophthalmology)
ICCM	idiopathic congestive cardiomyopathy
ICCU	intensive coronary care unit
ICD	idiopathic cerebral dysfunction implantable cardioverter defibrillator instantaneous cardiac death International Classification of Diseases intrauterine contraceptive device
ICE	ice, compression, elevation
ICF	intensive care facility intermediate care facility intracellular fluid

ICG	indocyanine green (dye)
ICH	infantile cortical hyperostosis intracerebral hemorrhage intracranial hemorrhage
ICJ	ileocecal junction
ICLE	intracapsular lens extraction
ICM	intercostal margin
ICN	intensive care nursery intercostal neuralgia
ICP	intracranial pressure
ICPC	intracranial pressure catheter
ICPMM	incisors, canines, premolars, molars
ICPP	intubated continuous positive pressure
ICR	intrastromal corneal ring
ICS	intercostal space intermediate coronary syndrome intracranial stimulation
ICSH	interstitial cell-stimulating hormone (laboratory/endocrinology)
ICT	indirect Coombs' test (laboratory/blood bank) inflammation of connective tissue insulin coma therapy intracranial tumor isovolumic contraction time (heart)
ict	icterus (jaundice)

ict ind	icterus index
ICU	infant care unit intensive care unit intermediate care unit
ICW	intracellular water
ID	identification immunodeficiency immunodiffusion inclusion disease infant deaths infectious disease infective dose injected dose initial diagnosis initial dose internal diameter intradermal (injection site)
I & D	incision and drainage (operation/skin) irrigation and debridement (operation/skin)
IDA	image display and analysis iron deficiency anemia
IDAT	indirect antiglobulin test
IDD	insulin-dependent diabetes
IDDF	investigational drug data form
IDDM	insulin-dependent diabetes mellitus
IDDS	implantable drug delivery system
IDE	investigational drug exemption

IDI	induction-delivery interval
IDK	internal derangement of the knee
IDL	intermediate-density lipoprotein
IDM	infant of diabetic mother
IDP	initial dose period
IDR	intradermal reaction
IDS	immune deficiency state incremented dynamic scanning integrated delivery system
IDT	intradermal test
IDV	intermittent demand ventilation
IDVC	indwelling venous catheter
IE	infective endocarditis
I/E	inspiratory-expiratory ratio (pulmonary function test)
ie	that is (Latin: *id est*)
IEA	immunoenzyme assay intravascular erythrocyte aggregation
IEB	idiopathic erythroblastopenia
IEC	injection electrode catheter intraepithelial carcinoma
IEF	isoelectric focusing
IEL	intraepithelial lymphocytes

IEM	inborn error of metabolism
IEMG	integrated electromyogram (procedure/physical medicine)
IEOP	immunoelectroosmophoresis
IEP	idiopathic erythropoiesis immunoelectrophoresis intraesophageal pressure isoelectric point
IF	immunofluorescence inhibiting factor interferon interstitial fluid intrinsic factor involved field (radiology)
IFA	immunofluorescent assay indirect fluorescent antibody (laboratory test) interferon alpha
IFE	immunofixation electrophoresis
IFO	implanted fertilized ovum
IFR	infrared inspiratory flow rate (respiratory therapy)
IFV	intracellular fluid volume
IG	immune globulin immunology intragastric

Ig immunoglobulin (laboratory/serology)
Types of immunoglobulins:
IgA (gamma A)
IgD (gamma D)
IgE (gamma E)
IgG (gamma G)
IgM (gamma M)

IGDM infant of gestational diabetic mother

IGH idiopathic growth hormone

IGIV immune globulin, intravenous

IGR intrauterine growth retardation

IGT impaired glucose tolerance

IGV intrathoracic gas volume

IH infectious hepatitis
inguinal herniorrhaphy

IHA immune hemolytic anemia
indirect hemagglutination (laboratory/serology)

IHAS idiopathic hypertrophic aortic stenosis

IHB incomplete heart block

IHBT incompatible hemolytic blood transfusion

IHC idiopathic hemochromatosis
infantile hydrocephalus
intrahepatic cholestasis

IHD intrahepatic duct
ischemic heart disease

IHJ	intrahepatic jaundice
IHN	ischemic hemorrhagic necrosis
IHO	idiopathic hypertrophic osteoarthropathy
IHP	idiopathic hypopituitarism
IHPH	intrahepatic portal hypertension
IHR	intrinsic heart rate
IHSA	iodinated human serum albumin
(^{131}I)HSA	human serum albumin tagged with radioiodine (nuclear medicine)
IHSS	idiopathic hypertrophic subaortic stenosis in-home support services
IHT	insulin hypoglycemia test
II	icterus index image intensifier
IIA	indirect immunofluorescence assay (confirmation test for AIDS)
IICP	increased intracranial pressure
IICU	infant intensive care unit
IID	insulin-independent diabetes
IIE	ineffective idiopathic erythropoiesis
IIF	immune interferon indirect immunofluorescence
IIHR	insulin-induced hypoglycemic response

IJP	internal jugular pressure
IL-1, IL-2	interleukin-1, interleukin-2
ILA	insulin-like activity
ILBBB	incomplete left bundle branch block (ECG)
ILBW	infant, low birth weight
ILC	incipient lethal concentration (radiology)
ILD	interstitial lung disease ischemic leg disease ischemic limb disease
ILL	intermediate lymphocytic lymphoma
ILP	intraligamentary pregnancy
IM	impaired mentation infectious mononucleosis internal medicine intramedullary (orthopedics) intramuscular (injection site)
IMA	inferior mesenteric artery internal mammary artery (implant) (operation/heart)
IMAA	iodinated macroaggregated albumin
IMAG	internal mammary artery graft (heart bypass surgery)
IMB	intermenstrual bleeding
IMBC	indirect maximum breathing capacity (pulmonary function test)

IMC	irregular menstrual cycle
IMCA	intramural coronary artery
IME	independent medical examination
IMF	idiopathic mediastinal fibrosis intermaxillary fixation
IMH	idiopathic myocardial hypertrophy
IMI	inferior myocardial infarction
imm	immobility immunology
IMN	ischemic muscular necrosis
imp	impacted (dentistry) important impression improved
impx	impaction (dentistry)
IMR	Individual Medical Record infant mortality rate
IMS	inframammary syndrome
IMT	induced muscular tension
IMV	inferior mesenteric vein intermittent mandatory ventilation (respiratory therapy)
IN	insulin intranasal
In	inulin

inac	inactive
INC	image not clear inside-needle catheter
inc	incision incomplete incontinent increase incurred
incl	including
$IncO_2$	incubator oxygen
incr	increased increment
IND	investigational new drug (approved for human testing)
ind	independent indirect
indic	indication
INDM	infant of nondiabetic mother
inf	infant infantile infected inferior infusion
inf dis	infectious disease
Inf MI	inferior wall myocardial infarction
infx	infection

ing	inguinal
INH	isonicotinic acid hydrazide (isoniazid) (medication order)
inh	inhalation
inj	inject injury
INO	intranuclear ophthalmoplegia
inoc	inoculate
inop	inoperable
INPAV	intermittent negative-pressure assisted ventilation (respiratory therapy)
INREM	internal radiation dose
INS	idiopathic nephrotic syndrome
ins	insert insurance
INSK	interstitial nonsyphilitic keratitis
insol	insoluble
inspir	inspiration
inst	instrument
insuf	insufficient
int	internal
Int Med	internal medicine

intox intoxication

int rot internal rotation

inv inverse
involuntary

IO inferior oblique (muscle)
inoperable
internal os (cervix)
intestinal obstruction
intraocular

I & O intake and output (of fluids)

IOA intraoral appliance

IOC intern on call

IOD interorbital distance (ophthalmology)

IODM infant of diabetic mother

IOF intraocular fluid

IOFB intraocular foreign body

IOL induction of labor
intraocular lens

IOML infraorbitomeatal line

ION ischemic optic neuropathy

IOP intraocular pressure

IORT intraoperative radiotherapy

IOS intraoperative sonography

IOT	intraocular tension
IOV	initial office visit
IP	incubation period induction period (anesthesiology) initial pressure inpatient interphalangeal (joint) intraperitoneal (injection site) isoelectric point
I & P	influenza and pneumonia
IPA	isopropyl alcohol
IPB	intraperitoneal bleeding
IPCD	infantile polycystic disease
IPD	idiopathic Parkinson's disease intermittent peritoneal dialysis
IPE	initial psychiatric evaluation interstitial pulmonary emphysema
IPF	idiopathic pulmonary fibrosis
IPG	impedance plethysmography
IPGE	immunoreactive prostaglandin E
IPH	idiopathic pulmonary hemosiderosis
IPJ	interphalangeal joint
IPP	income protection plan (hospitalization) inflatable penile prosthesis intermittent positive pressure (respiratory therapy)

IPPA inspection, palpation, percussion, auscultation

IPPB intermittent positive pressure breathing (respiratory therapy)

IPPI interruption of pregnancy for psychiatric indication

IPPO intermittent positive pressure inflation with oxygen (respiratory therapy)

IPPV intermittent positive pressure ventilation (respiratory therapy)

IPR independent professional review

IPS initial prognostic score

IPSP inhibitory postsynaptic potential

IPSS infantile partial striatal sclerosis

IPT intermittent pelvic traction

IPTH immunoreactive parathyroid hormone

IPU inpatient unit

IPV inactivated poliomyelitis vaccine

IQ intelligence quotient

IR immune response
immunoreactive
inconclusive results
inferior rectus (muscle)
infrared rays (procedure/physical medicine)
insulin resistance

IR *(cont)* internal resistance
internal rotation (orthopedics)
irritant reaction

IRB institutional review board (hospital)

IRBBB incomplete right bundle branch block (ECG)

IRC inspiratory reserve capacity

IRDS idiopathic respiratory distress syndrome

IRI immunoreactive insulin

IRMA immunoradiometric assay

IRP immunoreactive proinsulin

IRR intrarenal reflux

irr irradiation

irrig irrigation

IRS India rubber skin
infrared spectrophotometry

IRSA idiopathic refractory sideroblastic anemia

IRT isometric relaxation time (orthopedics)

IRV inspiratory reserve volume
(pulmonary function test)

IS immune serum
induced sputum
in situ (in original place)
intercostal space
interspace
intraspinal

I & S	indomethacin and spironolactone
ISA	intrinsic sympathomimetic activity iodinated serum albumin
ISC	insoluble collagen interstitial cells irreversible sickle cells
ISD	inhibited sexual drive initial sleep disturbance
ISDN	isosorbide dinitrate
ISE	ion-selective electrode
ISF	interstitial fluid
ISG	immune serum globulin (medication order)
ISH	icteric serum hepatitis
ISI	injury severity index (emergency medicine)
isol	isolation
isom	isometric
ISP	interstitial pregnancy
ISR	information storage and retrieval
IS10S	10% invert sugar in saline
IST	insulin sensitivity test (laboratory/endocrinology) insulin shock therapy (procedure/psychiatry)
ISW	interstitial water

IS10W	10% invert sugar in water
IT	inhalation therapy (respiratory therapy) intensive therapy (rehabilitation) intertuberous (pelvic diameter) intradermal test intrathoracic intratracheal intratracheal tube
ITFF	intertrochanteric femoral fracture
ITFS	incomplete testicular feminization syndrome
ITFx	intertrochanteric fracture
Ith	intrathecal (intraspinal)
ITP	idiopathic thrombocytopenic purpura interim treatment plan
ITT	insulin tolerance test (laboratory/endocrinology)
ITX	intertriginous xanthoma
IU	International Unit intrauterine
IUC	idiopathic ulcerative colitis
IUCD	intrauterine contraceptive device
IUD	intrauterine death intrauterine device
IUFB	intrauterine foreign body
IUFD	intrauterine fetal distress

IUGR	intrauterine growth rate intrauterine growth retardation
IUH	initial urinary hesitancy
IU/L	International Units per liter
IUP	intrauterine pregnancy
IUPC	intrauterine pressure catheter
IV	interventricular (heart) intervertebral intravascular intravenous
IVAC	intravenous automated controller
IVBH	intraventricular brain hemorrhage
IVC	inferior vena cava inspired vital capacity intravenous cholangiogram (x-ray/gallbladder)
IVCC	intravascular consumption coagulopathy
IVCD	intraventricular conduction defect (ECG)
IVCP	inferior vena cava pressure
IVCU	isotope-voiding cystourethrogram
IVCV	inferior venacavography (x-ray/vascular)
IVD	insufficient ventilatory drive intervertebral disc
IVDA	intravenous drug abuser

IVDSA	intravenous digital subtraction angiography
IVDU	intravenous drug user
IVF	intravascular fluid intravenous fluid in vitro fertilization (gynecology)
IVGTT	intravenous glucose tolerance test (laboratory/endocrinology)
IVH	intravenous hyperalimentation intraventricular hemorrhage (brain)
IVHT	intravenous histamine test (allergy)
IVIG	intravenous immunoglobulin
IVJC	intervertebral joint complex
IVLBW	infant of very low birth weight
IVNTG	intravenous nitroglycerin (medication order)
IVOX	intravascular oxygenator
IVP	intravenous push (dose) intravenous pyelogram (x-ray/kidneys) intraventricular pressure
IVPB	intravenous piggyback (infusion)
IVPF	isovolume pressure flow
IVR	idioventricular rhythm (cardiology)
IVSD	interventricular septal defect (heart)

IVT	intravenous transfusion
IVTTT	intravenous tobutamide tolerance test
IVU	intravenous urogram (x-ray/kidneys)
IVV	intravenous vasopressin
IW	ideal weight
IWI	inferior wall infarction
IWL	infant water loss
IWMI	inferior wall myocardial infarction
IWT	impacted wisdom teeth
IZS	insulin zinc suspension

J

J	Jewish joint joule (electrical measurement) juvenile
J1, J2, J3	Jaeger test (types 1-3) (ophthalmology)
JA	joint aspiration
JABE	juxtaarticular bone erosion
JAR	juvenile alveolar rhabdomyosarcoma
JBE	Japanese B encephalitis
JC	joint contracture
jc	juice (diet order)
JCF	juvenile calcaneal fracture
jct	junction
JD	jejunal diverticulitis
JDM	juvenile diabetes mellitus
jej	jejunum
JEV	Japanese encephalitis virus
JF	joint fluid
JFS	jugular foramen syndrome
jg	jugular
JGA	juxtaglomerular apparatus (kidney)

JGC	juxtaglomerular cell (kidney)
JGI	jejunogastric intussusception
JI	jejunoileostomy
JIB	jejunoileal bypass
JJ	jaw jerk (neurologic examination)
JKP	jackknife position (urology)
JLO	jejunal loop obstruction
JLP	juvenile laryngeal papilloma
JMD	juvenile macular degeneration
JND	just noticeable difference
jnd	jaundice
JOD	juvenile-onset diabetes
JPA	juvenile paralysis agitans (parkinsonism)
JPB	junctional premature beat
JPC	junctional premature contraction
JPD	Jackson-Pratt drain
JR	junctional rhythm
JRA	juvenile rheumatoid arthritis
JS	joint space
JSMA	juvenile spinal muscular atrophy

JT	jejunostomy tube
jt	joint (orthopedics)
JV	jugular vein
JVC	jugular venous catheter
JVD	jugular venous distention
JVP	jugular venous pulse
JVPT	jugular venous pulse tracing
JW-NT	Jehovah's Witness — no transfusions
JXG	juvenile xanthogranuloma

K

K	absolute zero (temperature) dissociation constant electrostatic capacity equilibrium constant kanamycin (on culture and sensitivity reports) Kelvin (temperature) kidney kilogram permeability coefficient potassium (Latin: *kalium*) (laboratory/chemistry) thousand (kilo)
k	rate (velocity) constant
17K	17-ketosteroid excretion (laboratory/endocrinology)
KA	ketoacidosis
K/A	ketogenic-antiketogenic ratio
KAC	kidney adenocarcinoma
KAF	kidney arteriovenous fistula
KAFO	knee-ankle-foot orthosis
KAS	Katz Adjustment Scale (psychiatry)
KB	ketone bodies (laboratory/urine) knee brace knuckle-bender (splint) Kussmaul breathing
K/B	knee-bearing (prosthesis)

KC	keratoconjunctivitis
K/C	knees to chest
kc	kilocycle (electrical measurement)
kcal	kilocalorie
KCCT	kaolin-cephalin clotting time
KCF	key clinical findings
KCG	kinetocardiogram
KCl	potassium chloride (medication orders/prescriptions)
KCP	knee-chest position
KCS	keratoconjunctivitis sicca
kc/s	kilocycles per second
KD	kidney donor knee disarticulation
KDA	known drug allergies
kDa	kilodalton
KDT	knee-drop test (orthopedics)
K_e	exchangeable body potassium
KED	Kendrick extrication device
KEP	knee-elbow position
keto	17-ketosteroid (laboratory/endocrinology)

kev	kiloelectron volts
KF	kidney failure
KFAB	kidney-fixing antibody
KFn	kidney function
KFS	Klippel-Feil syndrome
kg	kilogram
kG	kilogauss
kg/cal	kilogram-calorie
KGS	ketogenic steroid (laboratory/endocrinology)
KHF	Korean hemorrhagic fever
KHG	ketotic hyperglycinemia (neonatology)
KICB	killed intracellular bacteria
KID	keratitis, ichthyosis, deafness (syndrome)
kilo	kilogram (1000 grams)
KJ	knee jerk (neurologic examination)
KK	knee kick (neurologic examination)
KKK	Kolmer-Kline-Kahn (syphilis test)
kl	kiloliter
KLB	Klebs-Loeffler bacillus (on bacteriology reports)

Klebs	Klebsiella (on bacteriology reports)
KLS	kidney, liver, spleen Kleine-Levine syndrome (psychiatry)
KM	kanamycin (on culture and sensitivity reports)
km	kilometer
KMA	kinetic motor aphasia
km/s	kilometers per second
KMSV	Kirsten murine sarcoma virus
KMV	killed measles-virus vaccine
kn	knee
KNO	keep needle open
K/O	keep open
KP	keratitic precipitate keratitis punctata (eye examination)
KPR	key pulse rate
KPV	killed parenteral vaccine
KRP	Krebs-Ringer phosphate (intravenous solution)
KRRS	kinetic resonance Raman spectroscopy
KRT	kineradiotherapy

KS	Kaposi's sarcoma ketosteroid (laboratory/endocrinology) kidney stone Klinefelter's syndrome kyphoscoliosis
KSP	kidney-specific protein
KT	kidney transplantation
KTRP	Kolmer test with Reiter protein
KTU	kidney transplant unit
KUB	kidney, ureter, bladder (x-ray/urology)
KUF	kidney ultrafiltration rate
KUS	kidney, ureter, spleen (x-ray/urology)
KV	killed virus
kva	kilovolt-ampere
KVO	keep vein open (intravenous therapy)
kvp	kilovolt peak
KW	Keith-Wagener (eyeground findings) Kimmelstiel-Wilson (disease)
kw	kilowatt
KWB	Keith-Wagener-Barker (classifications of eyeground findings)
kyf	kyphosis

L

L	lateral left length lidocaine ligament lingual (surface) liter lower lumbar lumen lung
Ⓛ	left
l	line long loose
L_1, L_2...	lumbar vertebrae 1, 2...
LA	lactic acid (laboratory/chemistry) large amount latex agglutination left arm left atrium left auricle let alone local anesthesia long-acting (drug)
L & A	light and accommodation (eye examination)
LAA	left atrial abnormality leukocyte ascorbic acid
lab	laboratory

LAC	left atrial contraction long arm cast
lac	laceration
lact	lactating
LAD	lactic acid dehydrogenase left anterior descending (coronary artery) left axis deviation
LADCA	left anterior descending coronary artery
LAE	left atrial enlargement
LAF	laminar air flow lymphocytic-activating factor
LAFB	left anterior fascicular block
LAG	lymphangiogram
LAH	left anterior hemiblock (ECG) left atrial hypertrophy
LAI	left atrial involvement leukocyte adherence inhibition (assay)
LAIT	latex agglutination inhibition test (laboratory/serology)
LAKC	lymphokine-activated killer cells
LAL	left axillary line
LAM	left atrial myxoma
Lam	laminectomy
LAN	lymphadenopathy

LAO	left anterior oblique
LAP	laryngeal adductor paralysis left atrial pressure leucine aminopeptidase leukocyte alkaline phosphatase (laboratory/hematology)
lap	laparoscopy (procedure/abdominal)
LAPMS	long arm posterior molded splint
lapt	laparotomy (operation/abdominal)
LAR	laryngology late asthmatic response left arm recumbent leukocyte automatic recognition
LAS	long arm splint lymphadenopathy syndrome
LASER	light amplification by stimulated emission of radiation (radiation therapy)
LASS	labile aggregation stimulating substance
LAST	leukocyte-antigen sensitivity test
LAT	latex agglutination test left anterior thigh (injection site)
lat	lateral
lat decub	lateral decubitis (x-ray/abdomen)
lat men	lateral meniscectomy (orthopedics)
LATS	long-acting thyroid stimulator

LAUP	laser-assisted uvulopalatoplasty
LAV	lymphadenopathy-associated virus
LAVH	laparoscopy-assisted vaginal hysterectomy
lax	laxative (medication order)
LAY	look after yourself
LAYH	look after your heart
LB	large bowel laser bullectomy left buttock (injection site) live birth loose body low back
lb	pound (Latin: *libra*)
L & B	left and below
LBB	left breast biopsy
LBBB	left bundle branch block (ECG)
LBCD	left border of cardiac dullness
LBF	localized bone fibrosis
LBH	length, breadth, height
LBL	lymphoblastic lymphoma
LBM	last bowel movement lean body mass
lBM	loose bowel movement

LBNP	lower body negative pressure
LBO	large bowel obstruction
LBP	low back pain low blood pressure
LBS	low back strain
LBT	lactulose breath test
LbT	lupus band test
LBVP	luminal balloon valvuloplasty
LBW	low birth weight
LC	late clamped (umbilical cord) lethal concentration (radiation) living children low-calorie
LCA	left carotid artery leukocyte common antigen localized cutaneous atrophy
LCAH	life care at home
LCC	laparoscopic cholecystectomy light-cured composite (restoration) (dentistry)
LCCA	left common carotid artery
LCCS	lower cervical cesarean section
LCFA	long-chain fatty acid
LCIS	lobular carcinoma in situ

LCL	lymphocytic leukemia
LCLD	low-calorie liquid diet
LCLS	lymphocytic lymphosarcoma
LCM	large case management left costal margin lymphocytic choriomeningitis
LCR	late cutaneous reaction (allergy)
LCS	low continuous suction
LCT	long-chain triglyceride lymphocytotoxicity test
LCx	left circumflex (coronary artery)
LCyA	left coronary artery
LD	laboratory data learning disability left deltoid (injection site) legionnaire's disease leukodystrophy light difference (eye examination) living donor loading dose longitudinal diameter low density low dose Lyme disease
L/D	light/dark ratio (ophthalmology)
L & D	labor and delivery
LD_{50}	median lethal dose

LDB	Leishman-Donovan bodies (laboratory/bacteriology)
LDC	leukocyte differential count
LDD	light-dark discrimination (eye examination)
LDH	lactate dehydrogenase (laboratory/chemistry)
LDL	low-density lipoproteins (laboratory/chemistry)
L-Dopa	levodopa (medication order)
LDR	labor, delivery, recovery
LDUB	long double upright brace
LE	left eye lower extremity lupus erythematosus
LED	lupus erythematosus disseminatus
LEEP	loop electrosurgical excision procedure (biopsy method)
LEM	lateral eye movements
LEP	lupus erythematosus preparation (laboratory/hematology)
LES	lower esophageal sphincter
LESS	lateral electrical spine stimulation (orthopedics)
leuko	leukocytes (laboratory/hematology)

lev	levator (muscle)
LEVT	lower extremity venous tracing
LF	latex fixation (test) (laboratory/serology) low forceps (delivery) low frequency
LFA	left femoral artery left forearm left frontoanterior (fetal position) low friction arthroplasty
LFD	lactose-free diet (diet order) low fat diet (diet order) low forceps delivery
LFH	left femoral hernia
LFl	latex flocculation test (laboratory/serology)
LFOV	large field of view (radiology)
LFP	left frontoposterior (fetal position)
LFS	liver function series (laboratory/chemistry)
LFT	left frontotransverse (fetal position) liver function tests
LG	laryngectomy left gluteus (injection site) lymph glands
lg	large
LGA	large for gestational age
LGB	Landry-Guillain-Barré (syndrome) lateral geniculate body

LGB *(cont)*	lazy gallbladder (biliary atony)
LGFD	looks good from doorway (patient unofficial status)
LGH	lactogenic hormone
LGL	large granular lymphocyte Lown-Ganong-Levine (syndrome)
LGN	lobular glomerulonephritis
LGV	lymphogranuloma venereum
LH	left hand luteinizing hormone (laboratory/endocrinology)
LHF	left heart failure
LHH	left homonymous hemianopsia
LHL	left hepatic lobe
LHP	left hemiparesis
LHQ	Life History Questionnaire
LHRH	luteinizing hormone releasing hormone
LHS	left heart strain
LHV	left hepatic vein
LI	left iliac (artery)
Li	lithium
LIA	leukemia-associated inhibitory activity

LIBC	latent iron-binding capacity
LIC	left iliac crest
LICA	left internal carotid artery
LICM	left intercostal margin
LICS	left intercostal space
LIF	left iliac fossa (injection site) leukocyte inhibitory factor
lig	ligament
LIH	left inguinal hernia
LIHA	low impulsiveness, high anxiety (psychiatry)
LIMA	left internal mammary artery
lin	linear liniment (medication orders/prescriptions)
LIP	lymphoid interstitial pneumonitis
LIQ	lower inner quadrant
liq	liquid (diet order)
liqr	liquor
LIRBM	liver, iron, red bone marrow
LIS	left intercostal space low intermittent suction
LISS	low-ionic-strength saline solution

lith	lithotomy
LIV	left innominate vein
LK	lamellar keratectomy left kidney
LKS	liver, kidney, spleen
LL	left lateral left leg left lower left lung lower lid lower lobe
LLA	lobar lung atrophy
LLB	long-leg brace (orthopedics)
LLC	long-leg cast (orthopedics)
LLD	left lateral decubitus (position)
LLE	left lower extremity
LLF	left lateral femoral (injection site)
LL-GXT	low-level graded exercise test
LLL	left lower lobe (lung)
LLM	localized leukocyte mobilization
LLO	Legionella-like organism
LLPMS	long-leg posterior molded splint
LLQ	left lower quadrant

LLR	left lateral rectus (eye muscle)
LLS	long-leg splint
LLSB	left lower sternal border
LLT	left lateral thigh (injection site)
LLWC	long-leg walking cast
LM	legal medicine light microscopy longitudinal muscle
L/M	left message
LMA	left mentoanterior (fetal position)
LMB	left mainstem bronchus
LMC	lymphocyte-mediated cytotoxicity
LMCA	left main coronary artery
LMCL	left midclavicular line
LMD	local medical doctor low-molecular-weight dextran (intravenous solution)
LMF	lymphocytic mitogenic factor
L/min	liters per minute
L/min/m^2	liters per minute per square meter
LML	left mediolateral (episiotomy) (operation/obstetrics)
LMM	lentigo malignant melanoma

LMN	lower motor neuron
LMND	lower motor neuron deficiency
LMP	last menstrual period left mentoposterior (fetal position)
LMT	left mentotransverse (fetal position) leukocyte migration technique
LMW	low molecular weight
LN	lymph node
LN_2	liquid nitrogen
LNB	lymph node biopsy
LNCs	lymph node cells
LNE	lymph node excision
LNMP	last normal menstrual period
LO	leave open (lesion, incision)
LOA	leave of absence left occiput anterior (fetal position)
LOC	laxative of choice level of care (nursing) level of consciousness loss of consciousness loss of coordination
LOH	length of hospitalization
LOM	left otitis media limitation of motion loss of motion

LOMS	left otitis media, suppurative
LOP	leave on pass left occiput posterior (fetal position)
LOPS	length of patient stay
LOQ	lower outer quadrant
LOR	lack of response loss of resistance
LOS	length of stay
LOT	left occiput transverse (fetal position)
lot	lotion (medication orders/prescriptions)
LOVA	loss of visual acuity
LOWBI	low-birth-weight infant
LP	latent period leukocyte-poor light perception (eye examination) lipoprotein low power (microscopy) low pressure low protein (diet order) lumbar puncture (procedure/hematology)
L/P	lactate-pyruvate ratio
LPA	latex particle agglutination left pulmonary artery low physical activity
LPC	laser photocoagulation
LPD	lipoprotein deficiency

LPD *(cont)*	lower partial denture low-protein diet
LPE	lipoprotein electrophoresis (laboratory/chemistry)
LPF	leukocytosis promoting factor low power field (microscopy)
LPFB	left posterior fascicular block
LPH	left posterior hemiblock (ECG)
LPICA	left posterior internal carotid artery
LPL	lipoprotein lipase
LPN	Licensed Practical Nurse
LPO	left posterior oblique light perception only (eye examination)
LPS	lipopolysaccharide lung perfusion scan
LPV	left portal vein left pulmonary veins
LQ	left quadrant
LQTS	long QT syndrome (ECG reports)
LR	labor room lateral rectus (muscle) light reaction
L & R	left and right
L→R	left to right

LRA	left renal artery
LRD	living related (organ) donor
LRE	leukemic reticuloendotheliosis
LRF	liver residue factor
LRH	luteinizing hormone-releasing hormone
LRI	lower respiratory infection
LRM	left radical mastectomy
LRQ	lower right quadrant
LRR	labyrinthine righting reflex
LRS	lactated Ringer's solution (intravenous solution)
LRT	lower respiratory tract
LRv	life review process (psychotherapy)
LS	left side limbic system liver and spleen low salt lumbosacral lymphosarcoma
L/S	lecithin-sphingomyelin ratio
LSA	left sacrum anterior (fetal position) left subclavian artery
LSA/RCS	lymphosarcoma-reticulum cell sarcoma
LSB	left sternal border

LSC	late systollic click
LSCA	left scapuloanterior (fetal position)
LSCP	left scapuloposterior (fetal position)
LSD	lysergic acid diethylamide
LSF	low saturated fat (diet)
LSG	low specific gravity
LSH	lymphocyte-stimulating hormone
LSHG	leucine-sensitive hypoglycemia
LSIL	low-grade squamous intraepithelial lesion
LSK	liver, spleen, kidneys
LSLF	low sodium, low fat
LSM	late systolic murmur
LSO	left salpingo-oophorectomy (operation/gynecology)
LSP	left sacrum posterior (fetal position)
LSPA	left stenotic pulmonary artery
LSS	life support station liver-spleen scan lumbar spinal stenosis
LST	lateral sinus thrombophlebitis left sacrum transverse (fetal position) leptospirosis, spirochetosis, toxoplasmosis
LSTL	laparoscopic tubal ligation

LSV	left subclavian vein
LSW	left-side weakness
LT	laboratory technician left thigh left triceps leukotriene Levin tube (for gastrointestinal suction) long-term low-tension lymphotoxin
lT	levothyroxine
lt	left light
LTA	laryngotracheal anesthesia
LTB	laryngotracheal bronchitis
LTC	long-term care
LTCS	low transverse cesarean section
LTCU	long-term care unit
LTF	lymphocyte transforming factor
LTH	luteotropic hormone
LTM	long-term memory
LTT	leucine tolerance test
L & U	lower and upper
LUC	large, unstained cells

LUE	left upper extremity
LUIS	low-dose urea in invert sugar
LUL	left upper lobe (lung)
LUO	left ureteral orifice
LUQ	left upper quadrant
LV	left ventricle live vaccine live virus lung volume
LVA	left ventricular aneurysm
LVD	left ventricular dysfunction
LVE	left ventricular enlargement
LVEDP	left ventricular end-diastolic pressure
LVEDV	left ventricular end-diastolic volume
LVEF	left ventricular ejection fraction
LVET	left ventricular ejection time
LVF	left ventricular failure
LVFP	left ventricular filling pressure
LVH	left ventricular hypertrophy
LVID	left ventricular internal dimension
LVIDP	left ventricular initial diastolic pressure
LVN	Licensed Vocational Nurse

LVO	left ventricular outflow left ventricular overactivity
LVOT	left ventricular outflow tract
LVP	left ventricular pressure
LVSV	left ventricular stroke volume
LVSW	left ventricular stroke work
LVSWI	left ventricular stroke work index
LVV	left ventricular volume
LW	lateral wall living will
L & W	living and well
LWCT	Lee-White clotting time
LX	local irradiation
lymphs	lymphocytes (laboratory/hematology)
lytes	electrolytes (laboratory/chemistry)
lzms	lysozymes

M

M	male malignant married mass mesial (surface) mix (prescriptions) molar monocyte (on white blood counts) month morphine mother muscle Muslim Mycobacterium myopia (eye examination)
m	median meter minim (1/60 of a dram, or one drop) (medication orders/prescriptions) minute murmur
M_1, M_2	mitral heart sounds (first, second)
m^2	square meters (of body surface)
MA	medical assistant membrane antigen mental age mitral anulus muscle activity
ma	milliampere
MAA	macroaggregated albumin
MABP	mean arterial blood pressure

MAbs	monoclonal antibodies
MAC	maximum allowable concentration midarm circumference minimum alveolar concentration mitral anulus calcification Mycobacterium avium complex (AIDS complication)
mac	macerate
MACC	methotrexate, adriamycin, cyclophosphamide, CCNU (lomustine)
MAD	maximum acid determination mind-altering drugs
MADRS	Medicare Automated Data Retrieval System
MAE	moves all extremities
MAF	macrophage activating factor minimum audible field
mag	large (Latin: *magnum*)
mag cit	magnesium citrate (laxative)
magnif	magnification
MAH	monocular asteroid hyalitis (ophthalmology)
MAHA	microangiopathic hemolytic anemia
MAI	Mycobacterium avium-intracellulare
MAL	midaxillary line

malig	malignant
MALT	mucosa-associated lymphoid tissue
M + AM	compound myopic astigmatism
mam	milliampere minute
MAMC	midarm muscle circumference
mand	mandible
manif	manifestation
manip	manipulation
MAO	maximal acid output monoamine oxidase
MAOI	monoamine oxidase inhibitor
MAoP	mean aortic pressure
MAP	mean arterial pressure medical assistance program minimum audible pressure muscle action potential
MARIA	macroaggregated radioiodinated albumin
MAS	Manifest Anxiety Scale (psychiatry) meconium aspiration syndrome mobile arm support
mas	milliampere second
masc	masculine
MASER	microwave amplification by stimulated emission of radiation

mass	massage
MAST	military anti-shock trousers multiple antigen simultaneous test
mast	mastectomy
MAT	Miller-Abbott tube (gastrointestinal suction) Motivation Analysis Test multifocal atrial tachycardia
MAV	minute alveolar volume
max	maxillary maximum
MB	methylene blue (dye) microbiology
6MB	six-meal bland diet (diet order)
MBC	maximum breathing capacity minimal bactericidal concentration
MBD	minimal brain dysfunction
MBE	may be elevated
MBF	myocardial blood flow
MBL	menstrual blood loss minimal bactericidal level
MBM	mother's breast milk
MBP	major basic protein mean blood pressure
MbR	morbidity rate

MBT	midbrain tremor mixed bacterial toxin
MC	mast cell (on blood smear) maximum concentration metacarpal (joint) miscarriage mixed cellularity myocarditis
mc	millicurie (radioactivity measurement)
M & C	morphine and cocaine (drug addiction)
MCA	main coronary artery monoclonal antibodies
mCA	middle cerebral artery
MCAF	monocyte chemotactic and activating factor
MCAR	mixed cell agglutination reaction
MCB	membranous cytoplasmic bodies
McB	McBurney's point (appendix)
MCC	mean corpuscular hemoglobin concentration
MCCU	mobile coronary care unit
MCD	marginal corneal dystrophy mean cell diameter medullary cystic disease metaphyseal chondrodysplasia
MCE	medical care evaluation

MCF	macrophage chemotactic factor myocardial contractile force
mcg	microgram
MCGN	mesangiocapillary glomerulonephritis
MCH	mean corpuscular hemoglobin muscle contraction headache
MCHC	mean corpuscular hemoglobin concentration
MCHS	maternal and child health services
MCI	mean cardiac index
MCKD	multicystic kidney disease
MCL	midclavicular line midcostal line modified chest lead (ECG) most comfortable (sound) level
MCLS	mucocutaneous lymph node syndrome
MCO	marked corneal opacity
MCP	managed care plan metacarpophalangeal (joint)
MCR	metabolic clearance rate
MCS	multiple chemical sensitivity (allergy)
mc/s	megacycles per second
MCT	mean circulation time mean corpuscular thickness medium-chain triglyceride

MCT *(cont)*	medullary carcinoma of the thyroid
MCTC	metrizamide computed tomographic cisternogram
MCTD	mixed connective tissue disease
MCU	mobile care unit maximum care unit
mcU	microunit (on laboratory reports)
MCV	mean corpuscular volume
mcv	mean cell volume
MD	macular degeneration manic depressive mean deviation Meckel's diverticulum medical doctor mentally deficient minimum dosage mitral disease (cardiology) movement disorder (neurology) muscular dystrophy myocardial disease (cardiology)
MDA	manual dilatation of the anus motor discriminative acuity right mentoanterior (fetal position)
MDC	Major Diagnostic Category minimum detectable concentration
MDD	major depressive disorder mean daily dose
MDF	myocardial depressant factor

MDFR	midexpiratory dynamic flow rate
MDH	medullary dorsal horn
MDI	metered dose inhaler multiple daily injections
MDM	mid-diastolic murmur
MDP	manic depressive psychosis maximum deliverable pressure right mentoposterior (fetal position)
MDQ	minimum deductable quantity
MDR	minimum daily requirement
MDR-TB	multiple-drug-resistant tuberculosis
MDS	milk drinkers' syndrome minimum data sheet myocardial depressant substance
MDSO	mentally disordered sex offender
MDT	right mentotransverse (fetal position)
MDUO	myocardial disease of unknown origin
MDV	multiple dose vial (prescriptions)
MDY	month, date, year
ME	macular edema male escutcheon maximum effort Medical Examiner middle ear
M/E	myeloid-erythroid ratio

MEA	multiple endocrine adenomatosis
meas	measurement
MEC	minimum effective concentration
MECG	maternal electrocardiogram
MED	median erythrocyte diameter minimal effective dose minimal erythema dose (radiation therapy) multiple epiphyseal dysplasia
med	median medical medium (bacteriology)
MEDLARS	Medical Literature Analysis and Retrieval System
med men	medial meniscectomy
MEDPAR	Medicare Provider Analysis and Review
MEDPRO	Medical Education Resources Program
med stern	medial sternotomy
meds	medications (medicines)
MEE	middle ear effusion
MEF	maximal expiratory flow
MEFR	maximum expiratory flow rate
MEG	magnetoencephalogram
MEI	middle ear infection

MEL	metabolic equivalent level
MELAS	mitochondrial myopathy, encephalopathy, lactic acidosis and stroke-like symptoms
MEM	macrophage electrophoretic migration minimum essential medium
memb	membrane
MEN	multiple endocrine neoplasia (syndrome)
MEOS	microsomal ethanol oxidizing system
MEP	mean effective pressure meperidine (Demerol) motor end-plate (orthopedics)
mEq	milliequivalent (on chemistry reports)
MER	mean ejection rate (cardiology) methanol extraction residue
MERP	medical expense reimbursement plan
MES	maintenance electrolyte solution maximal electroshock seizure
MESA	myoepithelial sialadenitis
mesc	mescaline
met	metallic metastatic
metab	metabolic
metas	metastasis

metHb	methemoglobin
metMb	metmyoglobin
METS	metabolic equivalents (in exercise programs)
MeV	megaelectron volts
mev	millielectron volts
MF	march fracture medium frequency Millipore filter (for intravenous therapy) Mycosis fungoides myocardial fibrosis
M/F	male-female ratio
M & F	mother and father
MFA	malaise, fatigue, anorexia
MFAT	multifocal atrial tachycardia
MFB	metallic foreign body
MFD	mandibulofacial dysostosis midforceps delivery (obstetrics) minimum fatal dose
mfd	microfarad (electrical measurement)
MFEM	maximal forced expiratory maneuver
MFLB	macrofollicular lymphoblastoma
MFM	maternal-fetal medicine

MFPVC	multifocal premature ventricular contraction
MFR	midexpiratory flow rate mucus flow rate myofascial release (physical therapy)
MFS	maxillofacial surgery medical fee schedule mitral first sound
MFT	muscle function test
MG	membranous glomerulopathy menopausal gonadotropin myasthenia gravis
Mg	magnesium
mg	milligram
mg%	milligrams percent milligrams per hundred milliliters
MGD	mixed gonadal dysgenesis
MGF	maternal grandfather
MGM	maternal grandmother
MGN	membranous glomerulonephritis
MGPS	Marcus Gunn pupil sign
$MgSO_4$	magnesium sulfate
MGUS	monoclonal gammopathy of uncertain significance
MGXT	multistage graded exercise test

MH	maintenance hemodialysis malignant hyperthermia marital history medical history menstrual history mental health
MHA	microangiopathic hemolytic anemia microhemagglutination (syphilis test)
MHA-TP	microhemoglobin test for Treponema pallidum
MHB	maximum hospital benefit
MHb	methemoglobin
MHC	major histocompatibility complex maximal hip circumference mental health center multiphase health checkup
M/hct	microhematocrit
MHD	maximum human dose minimum hemolytic dose
MHE	multiple hereditary exostosis
MHK	metaherpetic keratitis
MHP	maternal health program
MHR	maximum heart rate (during stress test)
MHST	multiphasic health screen test
MHx	medical history
MI	mental illness

MI *(cont)*	mitral insufficiency myocardial infarction
MIC	maternal and infant care medical intensive care minimum inhibitory concentration mobile intensive care
micro	microscopic (microscopy) microscopic findings (in urinary sediment)
MICU	medical intensive care unit mobile intensive care unit
MID	minimal inhibiting dose minimal infective dose multiple infant dementia
mid sag	midsagittal
MIF	macrophage-inhibiting factor melanocyte-inhibiting factor midinspiratory flow migration-inhibiting factor
MIFR	maximal inspiratory flow rate
MIG	Medicare-insured group
MIH	migraine interparoxysmal headache
millisec	millisecond
min	minimum minor minute
MIO	minimum identifiable odor
MIP	maximum inspiratory pressure

MIPS	myocardial isotopic perfusion scan
misc	miscarriage miscellaneous
MIT	metabolic intolerance test miricidial immobilization test
mit insuf	mitral insufficiency
mIU	milli-International Unit (1/1000 of International Unit)
MIVP	mean intravascular pressure
mixt	mixture (medication orders/prescriptions)
MJ	marijuana medial joint
MJI	mid-joint injury
MK	monkey kidney (cell culture)
ML	malignant lymphoma middle lobe (of lung) midline
ml	milliliter
M/L	monocyte-lymphocyte ratio
MLA	mesenteric lymphadenitis
MLAP	mean left atrial pressure
MLB	midline bar monaural loudness balance (audiology)
MLC	minimum lethal concentration

MLC *(cont)*	mixed leukocyte culture
MlC	mixed lymphocyte culture
MLD	minimum lethal dose
mLD	median lethal dose (radiation)
MLE	midline episiotomy
MLF	medial longitudinal fasciculus
MLG	membranous lupus glomerulonephritis
ml/min/m^2	milliliters per minute per square meter
MLN	mucocutaneous lymph node
MLOS	maximum length of stay
MLR	middle latency response (audiology) mixed lymphocyte reaction
MLS	maxillary lymphosarcoma mean life span
MLT	medical laboratory technician
mLT	median lethal time
MM	malignant melanoma mucous membrane multiple myeloma
mM	millimol (electrolyte measurement)
mm	millimeter murmurs (heart) muscles

mm^3	cubic millimeter
M & M	milk and molasses (enema) morbidity and mortality
MMC	migrating myoelectric complex (neurology)
MMD	mass median diameter
MME	movable major equipment
MMECT	multiple-monitored electroconvulsive therapy
MMFR	maximal midexpiratory flow rate (pulmonary function test)
MMG	mean maternal glucose
mmHg	millimeters of mercury (blood pressure)
MMIS	Medicaid Management Information System
mM/L	millimoles per liter
MMM	myelosclerosis with myeloid metaplasia
mmm (mμ)	millimicron (microscopy)
MMP	matrix metalloproteinase
MMPI	Minnesota Multiphasic Personality Inventory (psychological test)
mmpp	millimeters partial pressure
MMR	mass miniature radiography maternal mortality rate

MMR *(cont)*	measles, mumps, rubella (immunization) mouth-to-mouth resuscitation
MMT	manual muscle test
MMTP	methadone maintenance treatment program
MN	midnight motor neuron myoneural
M & N	morning and night
Mn	manganese (laboratory/chemistry)
MNCV	motor nerve conduction velocity (procedure/physical medicine)
MND	maxillonasal dysplasia minimum necrotizing dose motor neuron disease
MNG	multinodular goiter
MNJ	myoneural junction
MNL	mononuclear leukocytes
MNP	malignant neoplasm
MO	medical officer mineral oil (medication order) minute output (of heart) months old
MO_2	myocardial oxygen
MOA	mechanism of action mechanism of allergy

MOB	maintenance of benefits (plan)
mob	mobile
MOC	maximum oxygen consumption multiple osteochondromatosis
MOD	maturity-onset diabetes
mod	moderate modified
MODS	multiple organ dysfunction syndrome
MOF	multiple organ failure
MOJAC	mood, orientation, judgment, affect, content
mol wt	molecular weight
MOM	milk of magnesia
mon	monocyte
Mono	infectious mononucleosis
mono	monocyte (laboratory/hematology)
MOP	medical outpatient program
MOPP	mechlorethamine, oncovin, procarbazine and prednisone (chemotherapy)
MOPV	monovalent oral poliovirus vaccine
MOR	monthly operating report
morph	morphine morphology

mort	mortality
MOSF	multiorgan system failure
mOsm	milliosmol
MOTT	mycobacteria other than tubercle (atypical tuberculosis)
MP	mean pressure mechanical percussion melting point menstrual period monophosphate multiparous
6-MP	6-mercaptopurine (medication order)
MPA	main pulmonary artery multiple progressive angioma
MPAP	mean pulmonary artery pressure
MPB	male pattern baldness
MPC	maximum permissible concentration (radiation)
MPCD	metaphyseal chondrodysplasia
MPCWP	mean pulmonary capillary wedge pressure
MPD	maximum permissible dose (radiation) mucopurulent discharge multiple personality disorder (psychiatry) myofacial pain dysfunction
MPDE	maximum permissible dose equivalent (radiation)

MPGN	membranoproliferative glomerulonephritis
MPHR	maximum predicted heart rate
MPI	maximun permitted intake (diet) maximum point of impulse (cardiology) multiphasic personality inventory (psychological test)
MPL	maximum permissible level (radiation)
MPP	maximum perfusion pressure
MPS	macular photocoagulation study mucopolysaccharide (with drug order)
MPV	mean platelet volume
MR	magnetic resonance may repeat medial rectus medical record mental retardation metabolic rate mitral reflux mitral regurgitation Moro reflex mortality rate
M & R	measure and record
MRA	magnetic resonance angiography medical record administrator
mrad	millirad
MRAP	mean right atrial pressure
MRBF	mean renal blood flow

MRD	medical record department minimal residual disease minimum reacting dose
MRE	maximum restrictive exercise
MRF	mitral regurgitant flow
MRFT	modified rapid fermentation test
MRG	median rhomboid glossitis murmurs, rubs, gallops (cardiology)
MRGT	magnetic resonance guided therapy
MRH	melanocyte-releasing hormone
MRHD	maximum recommended human dose
MRI	magnetic resonance imaging
M & R/I & O	measure and record intake and output (fluids)
MRL	minimal response level (radiation)
mRNA	messenger ribonucleic acid
MROC	malrotation of colon
MRS	magnetic resonance spectroscopy microaggregate recipient set
MRSA	methicillin-resistant Staphylococcus aureus
MRT	muscle response test
MRU	minimum reproductive units

MRV	minute respiratory volume
MRVP	mean right ventricular pressure
MR x 1	may repeat one time... (medication order)
MS	maladjustment score (psychiatry) maxillary sinus mental status minimal support mitral stenosis mucosubstance multiple sclerosis muscle strength musculoskeletal
MSA	mixed sleep apnea multiple system atrophy
MSAH	monosymptomatic adult hysteria (psychiatry)
MSAP	mean systemic arterial pressure
MSC	midsystolic click (cardiology)
MSCC	midstream clean catch (urine sample)
MSCL	mean sleep cycle length
MSD	midsleep disturbance multiple sulfatase deficiency
msec	millisecond
MSER	mean systolic ejection rate
MSET	multistage exercise test
MSG	massage

MSG *(cont)*	monosodium glutamate
MSH	melanocyte-stimulating hormone
MSI	motor-sensory impairment
MSK	medullary sponge kidney
MSL	midsternal line
MSLT	multiple sleep latency test
MSO_4	morphine sulfate
MSOF	multisystem organ failure
MSPs	multiple sexual partners
MSRPP	Multidimensional Scale for Rating Psychiatric Patients
MSS	mental status schedule muscular subaortic stenosis mucus-stimulating substance
MST	mean survival time (oncology)
M & ST	menthol and salicylamide tests (diagnostic procedure)
MSU	medical-surgical unit
msu	midstream urine (specimen)
MSUD	maple syrup urine disease
MSV	maximal sustained ventilation murine sarcoma virus
MSW	multiple stab wounds

MT	empty malignant teratoma mammary tumor massage therapy maximal therapy medial thickening metatarsal (joint) milieu therapy (Alzheimer's disease) muscle therapy muscle tone Mycobacterium tuberculosis
M/T	masses or tumors
MTBF	mean time between (systemic) failures
MTC	maximum toxic concentration medullary thyroid carcinoma
MTD	maximum tolerated dose metastatic trophoblastic disease
MTF	maximum terminal flow
MTI	minimum time interval
MTP	mesencephalic tegmental paralysis metatarsal periostitis metatarsophalangeal (joint)
MTR	mass, tenderness, rebound (abdominal examination)
MTT	maximal treadmill test mean transit time (cardiology)
MTU	methylthiouracil
MTV	mammary tumor virus

MTX	methotrexate (cancer chemotherapy)
MU	mouse unit (with reference to gonadotropins)
mu (μ)	micron (microscopy measurement)
MUC	maximum urinary concentration mucosal ulcerative colitis
MUGA	multigated angiogram
multip	multiparous
MUO	myocardiopathy of unknown origin
MUP	motor unit potential (neurology)
musc	muscles (muscular)
MUST	medical unit self-contained and transportable
MV	mechanical ventilation megavolts minute volume mitral valve mixed venous (blood)
mv	millivolts
MVA	motor vehicle accident
MVB	mixed venous blood
MVC	maximum vital capacity
MVE	mitral valve echo

MVI	minimal visual impairment multivitamin infusion
MVO_2	myocardial oxygen consumption
MVP	mitral valve prolapse (syndrome)
MVPP	mustargen, vinblastine, procarbazine, prednisone (chemotherapy)
MVR	mitral valve replacement
MVRI	mixed vaccine respiratory infection
MVS	mitral valve stenosis
MVV	maximum voluntary ventilation (pulmonary function test)
MW	molecular weight muscle wasting
mW	milliwatt
mw	microwave
Mx	mastectomy
mx	mixture
My	myopia (eye examination)
Myco	Mycobacterium
myelo	myelocyte
MyG	myasthenia gravis
myo	myocardial

MyoD1	myogenic regulatory gene
MZ	monozygotic

N

N	nasal negative nerve neutrophil never nitrogen none normal number
NA	Narcotics Anonymous needle aspiration noradrenaline not admitted not applicable not available nuclear antigen nucleic acid nurse anesthetist nurse's aide
Na	sodium
NAA	no apparent abnormalities
NABS	normal abdominal bowel sounds
NAC	N-acetylcysteine
NaCl	sodium chloride (intravenous solution)
NAD	nicotinamide adenine dinucleotide no active disease no acute distress no apparent distress no appreciable disease normal axis deviation (ECG) nothing abnormal detected

NAF	Native American female
NAG	narrow angle glaucoma
NAH	neonatal adrenal hemorrhage
NAI	nonaccidental injury
NAM	Native American male
NAN	neuroasthenic neurosis
NAP	neutrophil alkaline phosphatase nonacute profile
NAR	nasal airway resistance nonarticular rheumatism
narc	narcotic
Na/reab	sodium reabsorption rate
NAS	no added salt (diet order)
NASA	not a surgical abdomen (surgical consultation)
NAT	no action taken not adequately treated
NB	needle biopsy newborn normoblast note well (Latin: *nota bene*)
NBA	nonweight-bearing ambulation (orthopedics)
NBC	nuclear, biological, chemical

NBI	no bone injury
NBM	no bowel movements nothing by mouth (diet order)
NBN	newborn nursery
NBS	no bacteria seen (microscopy) normal bowel sounds
NBTE	nonbacterial thrombotic endocarditis
NBTNF	newborn, term, normal female
NBTNM	newborn, term, normal male
NBW	normal birth weight
NC	nasal cannula neurologic check no caffeine no change noncontributory
N/C	no charge no complaints not completed
NCA	neurocirculatory asthenia
NC/AT	normocephalic and atraumatic (head examination)
NCB	No Code Blue (emergency medicine)
NCD	normal childhood disease not considered disabling
NCE	nonconvulsive epilepsy
NCF	night care facility

NCJ	needle catheter jejunostomy
NCP	normal chromosomal pattern nursing care plan
NCPG	nonchromaffin paraganglioma
NCPR	no cardiopulmonary resuscitation
NCS	noncoronary sinus
NCT	nerve conduction time
NCVS	nerve conduction velocity studies
ND	natural death neonatal death neoplastic disease nerve deafness neurotic depression no data no disease nondisabling normal delivery (obstetrics) normal development (neonatology) not detectable not detected not determined not diagnosed not done
N/D	no defects
$\mathbf{N_d}$	refractive index (eye examination)
NDA	new drug application no date available
NDC	National Drug Code (number)

NDE	near death experience
NDF	no disease found
NDI	nephrogenic diabetes insipidus
NDN	nondysplastic nevi (dermatology)
NDP	net dietary protein
NDTI	National Disease and Therapeutic Index
NDV	Newcastle disease virus
NDx	nondiagnostic
NE	Neomycin nerve excitability neurologic examination no effect norepinephrine not elevated not enlarged not evaluated not examined nursing educator
neb	nebulizer
NEC	necrotizing enterocolitis nephrogenic erythrocytosis not elsewhere classified
NED	no evidence of disease no expiration date normal equivalent deviation
NEEP	negative end-expiratory pressure (respiratory therapy)

NEFA	nonesterified fatty acids
neg	negative
NEMD	nonspecific esophageal motility disorder
NEP	negative expiratory pressure nephrology
NER	no evidence of recurrence nonionizing electromagnetic radiation
NERD	no evidence of recurrent disease
nerv	nervous
NET	nasoendotracheal tube nerve excitability test
NEU	neurology
neut	neutrophil
NF	Nafcillin National Formulary necrotizing fasciitis (galloping gangrene) no fracture none found nonfasting normal flow not found
NFAR	no further action required
NFCC	neighborhood family care center
NFCD	nonfatal coronary disease
NFL	nerve fiber layer

NFM	neurofibromatosis
NFP	natural family planning
NFSA	nonfamilial splenic anemia
NFT	no further treatment
NFTD	normal full-term delivery
NG	nasogastric (tube) new growth nitroglycerin
N/G	no good
ng	nanogram (same as millimicrogram)
NGF	nerve growth factor
NGO	nitroglycerin ointment
NGRI	not guilty by reason of insanity
NGT	nasogastric tube
NGU	nongonococcal urethritis
NH	nursing home
NH_3	ammonia
NHA	no histologic abnormalities
NH_4Cl	ammonium chloride
NHD	normal hair distribution
NHDI	neurohypophyseal diabetes insipidus

NHJ	nonhemolytic jaundice
NHL	non-Hodgkin's lymphoma
NHM	no heroic measures
NHP	nocturnal hyperphagia nursing home placement
NHPP	normal human pooled plasma
NHS	normal human serum
NI	no improvement no information not identified not isolated
NIA	no information available
NIAL	not in active labor (obstetrics)
NICU	neonatal intensive care unit
NID	no identifiable disease
NIDDM	noninsulin-dependent diabetes mellitus
NIHD	noise-induced hearing damage
NIP	negative inspiratory pressure
NIR	non-identified risk (AIDS)
NIRR	noninsulin-requiring remission
NIT	nasointestinal tube
nitro	nitroglycerin

NITTS	noise-induced temporary threshold shift
NIV	noninvasive
NJF	nasojejunal feeding
n/k	not known
NKA	no known allergies
NKC	natural killer cell
NKDA	no known drug allergies
NKDC	nonketotic diabetic coma
NKHA	nonketotic hyperosmolar acidosis
NKHG	nonketotic hyperglycinemia
n/l	normal limits
NLA	neuroleptanalgesia
NLD	nasolacrimal duct
NLE	normal life expectancy
NLF	nasolabial fold
NLL	nonleukemic lymphoma
NLP	no light perception
NLT	not later than no less than
NM	neuromuscular nitrogen mustard (chemotherapy)

NM *(cont)*	nonmotile nuclear medicine
n/m	not measured not mentioned
NMA	neurogenic muscular atrophy
NMC	nodular mixed-cell (lymphoma)
NMD	normal mental development
NMI	no middle initial
NML	nodular mixed lymphoma
NMM	nodular malignant melanoma
NMN	no middle name
NMP	normal menstrual period
NMR	nuclear magnetic resonance (imaging procedure)
NMRS	nuclear magnetic resonance spectrophotography
NMS	neuroleptic malignant syndrome
NMT	no more than
NN	nurses' notes
N & N	nephritis and nephrosis
NNA	nonneuronopathic amyloidosis
NND	neonatal death

NNO no new orders (on medical records)

NNRTI nonnucleoside reverse transcriptase inhibitor

NNS nonnutritive sucking (neonatology)

NNT neonatology

NO nitric oxide
nursing office

n/o none obtained
not operable

no number

NOA notice of admission (hospital)

noct at night (Latin: *nocte*)

NOE no observable effect

NOFTT nonorganic failure to thrive

NOMI nonocclusive mesenteric infarction

NON nape of neck

non rep do not repeat (Latin: *nonrepetatur*)

non segs nonsegmented neutrophils

NOR noradrenaline (norepinephrine)

NOS not otherwise specified

NOTT nocturnal oxygen therapy trial

NP	nasopharyngeal (nasopharynx) near point neuropathology neuropsychiatric new patient nitroprusside not performed not present nucleoprotein nurse practitioner nursing procedure
NPA	nasopharyngeal airway near point of accommodation (eye examination) no previous admission
NPB	nodal premature beat
NPC	nasopharyngeal culture near point of convergence (eye examination) nephrogenic polycythemia nodal premature contraction nonproductive cough no previous complaint
NPD	Niemann-Pick disease nonprescription drug
NPDR	nonproliferative diabetic retinopathy
NPF	normal pelvic findings
NPH	neutral protamine Hagedorn (insulin) no previous history normal pressure hydrocephalus
NPhx	nasopharynx

NPI	no present illness
NPJT	nonparoxysmal junctional tachycardia
NPL	no perception of light
NPM	neonatal-perinatal medicine
NPN	nonprotein nitrogen (laboratory/chemistry)
NPO	nothing by mouth (Latin: *non per os*)
NPRL	normal pupillary reaction to light
NPSG	nocturnal polysomnogram
NPT	neoprecipitin test normal pressure and temperature
NQWMI	non-Q-wave myocardial infarction
NR	do not repeat (Latin: *non repetatur*) nonreactive nonrebreathing (oxygen mask) no refill (prescriptions) no response normal range not readable not recorded nuclear radiology
N/R	not remarkable
nr	near
NRAM	neuroretinal angiomatosis
NRB	nonreportable birth
NRBC	nucleated red blood cells

NRC	normal retinal correspondence (eye examination) not routine care
NREM	nonrapid eye movement (sleep)
NRI	neutral regular insulin
nRNA	nuclear ribonucleic acid
NRR	note, record, report (medical records)
NRS	normal rabbit serum
NRTP	nucleus reticularis tegmenti pontis
NS	nephrosclerosis nephrotic syndrome nervous system neurologic signs neurosurgery nonspecific nonsymptomatic normal serum no specimen (no sample) not stated
N/S	normal saline (intravenous solution) not seen not significant (on laboratory reports)
NSA	normal serum albumin no salt added no serious (significant) abnormality
NSAID	nonsteroidal anti-inflammatory drug
NSC	no significant change

NSCD	nonservice connected disability
NS/CST	nipple stimulation/contraction stress test
NSD	nominal standard dose normal spontaneous delivery no significant defect no significant deviation no significant difference no significant disease
NSE	neuron-specific enolase
NSFTD	normal spontaneous full-term delivery
nsg	nursing
NSGCT	nonsiminomatous germ cell tumor
NSH	normal scalp hair
NSHD	nodular sclerosing Hodgkin's disease
NSILA	nonsuppressible insulin-like activity
NSO	Neosporin ointment
NSOM	nonsuppurative osteomyelitis
NSP	nasal speech pattern not specified
NSPVT	nonsustained polymorphic ventricular tachycardia
NSQ	not sufficient quantity (on laboratory reports)

NSR	nasoseptal repair normal sinus rhythm (heart) not seen regularly
NSS	normal saline solution
NSSP	normal size, shape and position
NST	neostigmine test nonstress test no sooner than nutrition support team
NSU	nonspecific urethritis
NSV	nonspecific vaginitis
NSVD	normal spontaneous vaginal delivery
NSVT	nonsustained ventricular tachycardia
NT	nasotracheal (tube) nontender not tested
N & T	nose and throat
NTD	neural tube defect (birth defect)
NTE	not to exceed (medication order)
NTG	nitroglycerin
NTGO	nitroglycerin ointment
NTL	no time limit (medication order)
NTMI	nontransmural myocardial infarction
NTN	nephrotoxic nephritis

NTP	nitroprusside
NTR	nutrition
NTS	nasotracheal suction nontropical sprue
NTV	nervous tissue vaccine
NU	name unknown
nuc	nucleated
nucl	nucleus
NUD	nonulcerous dyspepsia
NUG	necrotizing ulcerative gingivitis
NUN	nonurea nitrogen
NV	naked vision (eye examination) next visit nonvaccinated nonvenereal normal value (on laboratory reports) Norwalk virus
N & V	nausea and vomiting
NVA	near visual acuity (eye examination)
NVD	nausea, vomiting, diarrhea neck vein distention no venereal disease
NVE	neovascular edema
NVL	neurovisceral lipidosis

NVS	neurological vital signs
NVT	nerve, vein, tendon
NW	nicotine withdrawal
NWB	nonweight-bearing
nx	nourishment
NYD	not yet diagnosed
NYHA	New York Heart Association (precedes heart disease classification)
NYP	not yet published
NZ	enzyme

O

O	eye (Latin: *oculus*) none objective occiput occlusal (surface) open opium oral orbit output
Ⓞ	by mouth
O_2	oxygen
O2	both eyes (eye examination)
O_3	ozone
$\bar{o}$	without
OA	occipital artery occiput anterior (fetal position) opioid antagonist optic atrophy osteoarthritis Overeaters Anonymous oxalic acid
O & A	observation and assessment
OAA	optic atrophy ataxia oxaloacetic acid
OAAD	ovarian ascorbic acid depletion (test)
OAD	obstructive airway disease

OAF	open air factor osteocyte activation factor
OAG	open angle glaucoma
OAP	ophthalmic artery pressure oxygen at atmospheric pressure
OASH	obstructive asymmetrical septal hypertrophy
OAVD	oculoauriculovertebral dysplasia
OB	obstetrics occult blood open biopsy
OBD	organic brain disease
OB-GYN	obstetrics-gynecology
OBK	ocular band keratitis
obl	oblique
OBS	organic brain syndrome
obsd	observed
obst	obstruction
OC	on call Ondine's curse (pulmonary medicine) only child operative cholangiography oral contraceptive ostomy care oxygen consumed
O & C	onset and course

OCA	oculocutaneous albinism oral contraceptive agent
O_2 cap	oxygen capacity
OCB	olivocochlear bundle
occ	occasionally occlusion occupation occurrence
OCCM	open chest cardiac massage
OCD	obsessive-compulsive disorder
OCDM	oculocranioorbital dysraphia-meningocele
OCFS	ovarian cancer family syndromes
OCG	oral cholecystogram
OCHP	oculocutaneous hyperpigmentation
OCPD	occult constrictive pericardial disease
OCR	oculocardiac reflex
OCT	oral contraceptive therapy ornithine carbamoyltransferase oxytocin challenge test (obstetrics)
OCU	observation care unit
OCV	ordinary conversational voice
OCX	oral cancer examination
OD	Doctor of Optometry ocular dentistry

OD *(cont)*	on duty open drop (anesthesia) optical density outside diameter overdose (drugs) right eye (Latin: *oculus dexter*)
od	every day (medication orders/prescriptions) once daily (Latin: *omni die*)
ODA	right occiput anterior (fetal position)
ODC	oxygen dissociation curve
ODM	ophthalmodynamometry
ODP	right occiput posterior (fetal position)
ODS	oxygen desaturation
ODT	right occiput transverse (fetal position)
OE	on examination otitis externa
O & E	observation and evaluation
OEE	outer enamel epithelium
OER	oxygen enhancement ratio
OES	optical emission spectroscopy
OF	open fracture
OFC	occipital-frontal circumference (head)
OFD	object-to-film distance (radiology)

OFE	ovarian fibroepithelioma
off	office official
OFTT	organ failure to thrive
OG	optic glioma orogastric (feeding)
OGF	ovarian growth factor
OGI	osteogenesis imperfecta
OGR	Orlon graft replacement
OGTT	oral glucose tolerance test (diabetes detection)
OH	occupational history open heart (surgery) oral herpes oral hygiene orthostatic hypotension
OHA	oral hypoglycemic agents
OHCS	hydroxycorticosteroid
OHD	organic heart disease
OHDC	oxyhemoglobin dissociation curve
OHF	Omsk hemorrhagic fever overhead frame
OHI	oral hygiene instructions
OHL	oral hairy leukoplakia

OHM	optimal health maintenance
OHP	obese hypertensive patient oxygen under high pressure
OHS	obesity hypoventilation syndrome open heart surgery
OHT	overhead trapeze
OI	opportunistic infection osteogenesis imperfecta oxygen intake
OIH	ovulation-inducing hormone
oint	ointment
OIRD	object-to-image receptor distance (radiology)
OJ	orange juice (diet order) orthoplast jacket
OKAN	optokinesia after nystagmus
OKN	optokinetic nystagmus
OL	otolaryngology
ol	oil (prescriptions)
OLA	left occipital anterior
OLB	open lung biopsy
OLD	occupational lung disease
OM	occupational medicine osteomyelitis

OM *(cont)*	otitis media oxygen mask
om	every morning (Latin: *omni mane*)
OMA	oculomotor apraxia
OMCA	otitis media, catarrhal, acute
OMD	ocular muscular dystrophy organic mental disorder otomandibular dysostosis
OME	otitis media with effusion
OMI	old myocardial infarction
OML	orbitomeatal line
OMP	oculomotor paralysis
OMPA	otitis media, purulent, acute
OMSA	otitis media, suppurative, acute
OMSC	otitis media, suppurative, chronic
OMT	osteopathic manipulative therapy
OMVC	open mitral valve commissurotomy
OMVI	operating a motor vehicle (while) intoxicated
ON	office nurse oncology optic nerve orthopedic nurse
OND	other neurologic disease

ONP	operating nursing procedure osteoplastic nasal periostitis
ONTR	orders not to resuscitate
OO	oophorectomy osteoid osteoma
OOB	out of bed
OOC	out of control
OOF	owned and operated facility
OOM	onset of menarche
OOR	out of room
OP	occiput posterior old (previously seen) patient opening pressure operative procedure osteoporosis outpatient
op	operation
O & P	ova and parasites
OPA	organ procurement agency
OPB	outpatient basis
OPCU	outpatient care unit
OPD	optical path difference outpatient department
OPG	ocular plethysmography

OPH	ophthalmology
OPL	other party liability
OPLS	osteopathic lumbosciatalgia
OPP	oxygen partial pressure
opp	opposite
OPR	orbicularis pupillary reflex
OPS	outpatient service
OPT	orbital pseudotumor outpatient treatment
opt	optical optimum optional
OPV	oral poliovirus vaccine
OR	open reduction (orthopedics) operating room
O/R	oxidation/reduction
ORD	optical rotatory dispersion
ORE	oil retention enema
OREF	open reduction with external fixation
org	organic
ORIF	open reduction with internal fixation
orig	origin

ORL	otorhinolaryngology
ORN	operating room nurse
ORP	oxidation-reduction potential
ORR	otolith-righting reflex (neonatology)
ORS	orthopedic surgery
ORT	oral rehydration therapy
orth	orthopedic
ORW	Osler-Rendu-Weber syndrome
ORx	oriented
OS	by mouth (Latin: *os*) left eye (Latin: *oculus sinister*) opening snap (heart sound) oral surgery orthopedic surgery osteogenic sarcoma osteosclerosis
OSA	obstructive sleep apnea optic system assessment
OSAS	obstructive sleep apnea syndrome
O_2 sat	oxygen saturation
osm	osmotic
OSMF	oral submucous fibrosis
osmo	osmolality (on laboratory reports)
OsP	osmotic pressure

OT	occlusion time occupational therapy ocular tension (eye examination) olfactory threshold oral thrush orotracheal (tube) orthopedic traction otology
OTA	orthotoluidine ardenite (urology test)
OTC	over-the-counter (drugs) oxytetracycline
OTD	organ tolerance dose
OTO	otology
OTR	Registered Occupational Therapist
OTS	orotracheal suction
OU	both eyes together (Latin: *oculi unitas*) observation unit
OURQ	outer upper right quadrant (breast)
OV	office visit
Ov	ovary
O_2V	oxygen ventilation equivalent
OVAR	off-vertical axis rotation
OVD	occlusal vertical dimension (dentistry) oculovertebral dysplasia opticovestibular disturbance
OVX	ovariectomy

O/W	oil in water (medication base)
OWL	Old World leishmaniasis
OX	oxacillin
oxid	oxidized
OXT	oxytocin
OXZ	oxazepam
oz	ounce

P

P	parent parity (obstetrics) partial pressure (blood gases) penicillin percussion phosphorus (laboratory/chemistry) placebo plan plasma pressure private (patient or room) protein Protestant pulse pupil
^{32}P	radioactive phosphorus (nuclear medicine)
P1	first parental generation
P_1, P_2	pulmonic heart sounds (first, second)
p	mean (gas) pressure posterior
$\bar{p}$	after (Latin: *post*)
PA	panic attack paralysis agitans pernicious anemia physician's assistant plasma aldosterone posterior-anterior (chest x-ray) primary anemia prior to admission Professional Association prolonged action (tablets) pubic arch

PA *(cont)*	pulmonary artery pulsus alternans
P & A	percussion and auscultation
PAA	postantalgic atrophy
P(A-aDO_2)	alveolar-arterial oxygen tension difference
PAB	premature atrial beat
PABA	para-aminobenzoic acid
PABP	postalcoholic behavior pattern
PAC	phenacetin, aspirin, caffeine preadmission certification (hospital) premature atrial contraction
PACO_2	alveolar carbon dioxide tension
PaCO_2	arterial carbon dioxide tension
PACP	pulmonary artery counterpulsation
PACU	postanesthesia care unit
PAD	percutaneous abscess drainage peripheral arterial disease Pick's arteriopathic dementia primary affective disorder
PADP	pulmonary artery diastolic pressure
PAF	paroxysmal atrial fibrillation platelet activating factor pulmonary arteriovenous fistula
PAH	para-aminohippuric (acid) pulmonary artery hypertension

PAIg	platelet-associated immunoglobulin
PAL	posterior axillary line
palp	palpable
palpit	palpitations
PALS	periarteriolar lymphocyte sheath
PAM	phenylalanine mustard pulmonary alveolar microlithiasis
PAMP	pulmonary artery mean pressure
PAN	polyarteritis nodosa
PanX	panorex x-ray
PAO_2	alveolar oxygen partial pressure
PaO_2	arterial oxygen partial pressure
PAOP	pulmonary artery occlusion pressure
PAP	positive airway pressure primary atypical pneumonia private ambulatory patient pulmonary alveolar proteinosis pulmonary artery pressure
pAP	peak airway pressure
Pap	Papanicolaou smear (procedure/gynecology)
PA/PS	pulmonary atresia/pulmonary stenosis
PAR	perennial allergic rhinitis platelet aggregate ratio

PAR *(cont)*	possible allergic reaction postanesthetic recovery (room) pulmonary arteriolar resistance
para I, II	having borne one child, two children,...
par aff	to the part affected (Latin: *pars affecta*)
parent	parenteral (parenterally)
PAROM	passive assistive range of motion
part aeq	in equal parts (Latin: *partes aequales*)
PARU	postanesthetic recovery unit
PAS	para-aminosalicylic acid patient appointment and scheduling periodic acid-Schiff (stain) preadmission screening (hospital) pulmonary artery stenosis
PASP	pulmonary artery systolic pressure
pass	passive
PAT	paroxysmal atrial tachycardia plasma antithrombin preadmission testing (hospital) pregnancy at term
pat med	patent medicine
PAVF	pulmonary arteriovenous fistula
PAW	primary affective witzelsucht (neurology)
PAWP	pulmonary artery wedge pressure
PAX	periapical x-ray

PB	peripheral blood piggyback (intravenous administration) polymyxin B premature beats pressure breathing
Pb	lead (Latin: *plumbum*) presbyopia (eye examination)
pb	phenobarbital
P & B	phenobarbital and belladonna
PBA	percutaneous bladder aspiration
P_{BA}	brachial arterial pressure
PBAV	percutaneous balloon aortic valvuloplasty
PBC	peripheral blood cells primary biliary cirrhosis
PBD	percutaneous biliary drainage
PBF	pulmonary blood flow
PBG	porphobilinogen
PBI	protein-bound iodine (laboratory/endocrinology)
PBLI	premature birth, live infant
pbo	placebo
PBP	penicillin-binding protein porphyrin biosynthetic pathway progressive bulbar palsy
pBP	peak blood pressure

PBS	phosphate-buffered saline
PBSC	peripheral blood stem cell
PBV	predicted blood volume
PC	packed cells persistent condition platelet count portacaval (shunt) present complaint Professional Corporation pulmonary capillary
pc	after food (Latin: *post cibum*)
PCA	passive cutaneous anaphylaxis patient-controlled analgesia percutaneous carotid arteriogram plasma catecholamines
PCB	paracervical block (procedure/anesthesiology) percutaneous biopsy postcoital bleeding
PcB	near point of convergence to the baseline (eye examination)
PCC	patient care coordinator pheochromocytoma phosphate carrier compound primary care clinic
PCc	periscopic concave (eye examination)
PCCU	postcoronary care unit
PCD	phototoxic contact dermatitis plasma cell dyscrasia

PCD *(cont)*	polycystic disease postcoital depression precancerous dermatosis
PCE	precaliceal canalicular ectasia
PCF	prothrombin conversion factor
PCG	phonocardiogram (procedure/cardiology)
PCH	paroxysmal cold hemoglobinuria plasma cell hepatitis pseudochromhydrosis
PCI	pneumatosis cystoides intestinalis
pCi/L	picocuries per liter (radon measurement)
PCK	polycystic kidney (disease)
PCN	percutaneous nephrostomy
PCNA	proliferating cell nuclear antigen
PCNL	percutaneous nephrostolithotomy
PCO	patient complains of
pCO_2	partial pressure of carbon dioxide
PCOD	polycystic ovary disease
PCP	phencyclidine HCl (psychedelic drug "angel dust") Pneumocystis carinii pneumonia primary care physician pulmonary capillary pressure
PCR	polymerase chain reaction (DNA test) probable causal relationship

PCR *(cont)*	protein catabolic rate
P_{Cr}	plasma creatinine
PCS	patient care standards portacaval shunt (operation/liver) postcardiotomy syndrome pseudoclaudication syndrome (orthopedics)
PCT	paracentesis porphyria cutanea tarda portacaval transposition prism cover test prothrombin consumption test proximal convoluted tubule (kidney)
PCU	pain control unit palliative care unit protective care unit
PCV	packed cell volume parietal cell vagotomy polycythemia vera pressure control ventilation
PCW	pulmonary capillary wedge (pressure, tracing)
PCx	periscopic convex (eye examination)
PCXR	portable chest x-ray
PD	panic disorder Parkinson's disease patent ductus pediatrics peritoneal dialysis physical diagnosis poorly differentiated (cells) postural drainage

PD *(cont)* — pressor dose
progression of disease
psychotic dementia
pulmonary disease
pupillary distance

p/d — packs per day (cigarettes)

PDA — patent ductus arteriosus
pediatric allergy
pericardial diaphragmatic adhesion

PDC — pediatric cardiology
prolonged detention care

PDCE — precaliceal diffuse canalicular ectasia

PDD — progressive diaphyseal dysplasia

PDE — pediatric endocrinology

PDGF — platelet-derived growth factor

PDH — past dental history

PDN — private duty nurse

PDQ — pretty darn quick

PDR — pediatric radiology
Physician's Desk Reference

pdr — powder (medication orders/prescriptions)

PDS — pain dysfunction syndrome
postdiphtheritic stenosis
pediatric surgery

PDT — photodynamic therapy

PDU	pulsed Doppler ultrasonography
PDVP	permanent demand ventricular pacemaker
PDx	probable diagnosis
PE	panendoscopy pedal edema pharyngoesophageal physical examination plasma exchange pleural effusion psychotic episode pulmonary edema pulmonary embolism
P_E	expiratory pressure (respiration therapy)
PEARLA	pupils equal and react to light and accommodation
$PECO_2$	mixed expired carbon dioxide tension
PED	pre-existing disease progressive exertional dyspnea
PEEM	postexanthematous encephalomyelitis
PEEP	positive end expiratory pressure (respiration therapy)
pEF	peak expiratory flow
pEFR	peak expiratory flow rate
PEG	percutaneous endoscopic gastrostomy pneumoencephalogram (procedure/neurology)
PEI	phosphorus excretion index

PEM	probable error of measurement protein energy malnutrition
PEME	pulsed electromagnetic energy (diathermy)
PENG	photoelectric nystagmography
PENS	percutaneous epidural nerve stimulation
pent	pentothal
PEO	progressive external ophthalmoplegia
PEP	pre-ejection period (heart) protein electrophoresis (diagnostic procedure)
per	periodic
perf	perforation performed
periap	periapical
PERLA	pupils equal, react to light and accommodation
perm	permanent
perp	perpendicular
PERR	pattern-evoked retinal response
PERRLA	pupils equal, round, react to light and accommodation
pers	personal
PES	preexcitation syndrome (cardiology)

PES *(cont)*	programmed electrical stimulation (procedure/cardiology)
PESS	primary empty sella syndrome
PET	positron emission tomography pre-eclamptic toxemia psychiatric emergency team
PETF	proximal end tibial fracture
PETN	pentaerythrityl tetranitrate
PETT	positron emission transaxial tomography
peV	peak electron volts
PF	parenteral feeding peritoneal fluid plantar flexion platelet factor pulmonary function
PFB	present from birth
PFC	pelvic flexion contracture persistence of fetal circulation (syndrome) prefrontal cortex
PFFD	proximal femur focal deficiency
PFG	pelvic fat girdle porcelain fused to gold (dentistry)
PFI	percutaneous flank incision
PFK	phosphofructokinase photorefractor keratectomy (procedure/ophthalmology)

PFM	porcelain fused to metal (dentistry)
PFO	patent foramen ovale
PFP	platelet-free plasma
PFR	pleural friction rub
pFR	peak flow rate
P & FS	pit and fissure sealant (dentistry)
PFT	pulmonary function test
PFU	plaque-forming unit
PG	paregoric prostaglandin pyoderma gangrenosum
Pg	pregnant
pg	picogram (same as micromicrogram)
PgE	prostaglandin E (dinoprostone)
PgE_1	prostaglandin E_1 (alprostadil)
PGF	paternal grandfather
PGH	pituitary growth hormone
PgI_2	prostaglandin I_2 (prostacylin)
PGM	paternal grandmother
PGN	proliferative glomerulonephritis
PGU	postgonococcal urethritis

PH	past history personal history pin hole (eye examination) primary hypogonadism prostatic hypertrophy public health pulmonary hypertension
pH	hydrogen ion concentration power of hydrogen
PHA	passive hemagglutination phytohemagglutinin (laboratory/serology) pseudohypoaldosteronism
phar	pharmacy
PHC	posthospital care primary hepatic carcinoma
PHDD	personal history of depressive disorders
PHEN	pigmented hairy epidermal nevus (dermatology)
pheno	phenotype
pheo	pheochromocytoma
PHGG	polyclonal hypergammaglobulinemia
PHH	posthemorrhagic hydrocephalus
PHI	private health insurance
PHL	Philadelphia chromosome
PHMD	pseudohypertrophic muscular dystrophy

PHN	postherpetic neuralgia Public Health Nurse
PHO	pediatric hematology/oncology physician-hospital organization
phos	phosphate
PHP	prepaid health plan pseudohypoparathyroidism
PHPT	primary hyperparathyroidism
PHT	passive hyperimmune therapy peroxide hemolysis test phenylhydantoin pulmonary hypertension
PHTN	portal hypertension
phys	physical
phys dis	physical disability
PHx	past history
Phx	pharynx
PI	peripheral iridectomy (operation/ophthalmology) present illness primary infarction protease inhibitor pulmonary infarction
P_I	inspiratory pressure (respiratory therapy)
PIA	plasma insulin activity (laboratory/endocrinology)

PIAD	papular infantile acrodermatitis
PIC	preinvasive cancer
PICC	peripherally inserted central catheter
PICU	pediatric intensive care unit pulmonary intensive care unit
PID	pelvic inflammatory disease prolapsed intervertebral disc
PIDRA	portable insulin dosage regulating apparatus
PIE	pulmonary infiltration with eosinophilia pulmonary interstitial emphysema
PIEM	postinfective encephalomyelitis
pIFR	peak inspiratory flow rate (respiratory therapy)
PIFT	platelet immunofluorescence test
PIGN	postinfective glomerulonephritis
PIGPA	pyruvate, inosine, glucose, phosphate, adenine
PIH	pregnancy-induced hypertension primary intracerebral hemorrhage
PINS	person in need of supervision
pIP	peak inspiratory pressure postinspiratory pressure
PIPJ	proximal interphalangeal joint

PIT	picture identification test (psychiatry)
pit	pituitary
PITR	plasma iron turnover rate
PIVD	protruded intervertebral disc
PIVI	postirradiation vascular insufficiency
PIVR	pacemaker-induced ventricular rate
PIW	proposed ideal weight
PJB	premature junctional beat (ECG)
PJC	premature junctional contraction (ECG)
PJRT	permanent junctional reciprocating tachycardia
PJT	paroxysmal junctional tachycardia
PJVT	paroxysmal junctional ventricular tachycardia
PK	Prausnitz-Küstner (reaction) pyruvate kinase (assay)
pK	dissociation constant
PKD	polycystic kidney disease
PKU	phenylketonuria
PL	perception of light (eye examination) phospholipid placental lactogen
pl	place

pl *(cont)*	plasma
P_L	transpulmonary pressure
PLA	peroxidase-labeled antibodies (test)
PLD	pregnancy, labor, delivery
PLE	polymorphous light eruption
PLED	periodic lateralized epileptiform discharge
PLG	plasminogen proliferative lupus glomerulonephritis
PLI	professional liability insurance
PLMD	periodic limb movement disorder (sleep disorder)
PLOM	papillomatosis of lips and oral mucosa
PLP	pharyngolaryngeal paralysis
PLR	pronation/lateral rotation (orthopedics)
PLS	primary lateral sclerosis
PLT	platelets (laboratory/hematology)
PM	after death (Latin: *post mortem*) after noon (Latin: *post meridian*) night pacemaker petit mal (seizures) physical medicine pneumomediastinum polymorphs (white blood cells) presystolic murmur preventive medicine

PMA	progressive muscular atrophy
pMA	peroneal muscular atrophy
PMB	postmenopausal bleeding
PMC	percutaneous mitral commissurotomy pseudomembranous colitis
PMD	primary myocardial disease progressive muscular dystrophy
PME	postmenopausal estrogen (therapy)
PMF	progressive massive fibrosis
PMH	past medical history
PMI	past medical illness patient medication instructions point of maximum impulse point of maximum intensity postmyocardial infarction private medical insurance
PML	polymorphonuclear leukocyte progressive multifocal leukoencephalopathy
PMNs	polymorphonucleocytes
PMO	postmenopausal osteoporosis
PMP	pain management program past menstrual period
PMR	physical medicine and rehabilitation polymyalgia rheumatica proton magnetic resonance

PMRB	postmenopausal recurrent bleeding
PMS	pectoralis major syndrome postmenopausal syndrome premenstrual syndrome
PMT	premenstrual tension
PMTH	premenstrual tension headache
PMV	prolapsed mitral valve
PMW	progressive muscle weakness proximal muscle wasting
PN	parenteral nutrition peripheral nerve peripheral neuropathy polyarteritis nodosa postnatal
Pn	pneumonia
P & N	psychiatry and neurology
PNA	perinatal assessment
$\mathbf{P}_{\mathbf{Na}}$	plasma sodium
PNB	prostatic needle biopsy
PNC	premature nodal contraction
PND	paroxysmal nocturnal dyspnea postnasal drip
PNE	pneumoencephalography plasma norepinephrine

PNF proprioceptive neuromuscular facilitation (rehabilitation technique)

PNH paroxysmal nocturnal hemoglobinuria

PNI peripheral nerve injury
postnatal infection

PNLB percutaneous needle liver biopsy

PNM perinatal mortality

PNMA progressive neuromuscular atrophy

PNP pediatric nephrology
Pediatric Nurse Practitioner
peripheral neuropathy
psychogenic nocturnal polydipsia

PNPR positive-negative pressure respiration

PNS parasympathetic nervous system
paretic neurosyphilis
partial nonprogressing stroke
peripheral nervous system

PNT percutaneous nephrostomy tube

PO parietooccipital
postoperative

P/O phone order

P_o opening pressure

po by mouth (Latin: *per os*)

pO_2 partial pressure of oxygen

PO_4	phosphate
POA	point of application primary optic atrophy
POAG	primary open-angle glaucoma
POB	place of birth (medical records)
POBS	passage of bloody stool
POC	postoperative care postoperative check products of conception
POD	place of death (medical records) postoperative day postovulatory day
PODS	passage of dark stool
PODx	preoperative diagnosis
POE	periorbital edema point of entry (gunshot)
POEx	point of exit (gunshot) postoperative exercise
POF	pyruvate oxidation factor
POFO	passage of foreign object
POHA	preoperative holding area
POI	point of insertion
poik	poikilocytosis (of blood cells)
polio	poliomyelitis

POLS	passage of light stool
polys	polymorphonuclear leukocytes
POMP	prednisone, oncovin, methotrexate and 6-mercaptopurine (chemotherapy)
POMR	problem-oriented medical record
POP	plasma osmotic pressure plaster of Paris
pop	popliteal
POQU	procedure of questionable usefulness
POR	physician of record problem-oriented record
PORP	partial ossicular replacement prosthesis
PORR	postoperative recovery room
PORT	postoperative respiratory therapy
POS	polycystic ovary syndrome
pos	position positive
poss	possible
post	posterior postmortem
postop	postoperative
POU	placenta, ovaries, uterus
PP	positive pressure

PP *(cont)*	postpartum postprandial private patient proximal phalanx pulsus paradoxus (cardiology)
P & P	prothrombin-proconvertin (test)
pp	near point of accommodation (eye examination) pin prick pulse pressure
PPA	palpitation, percussion, auscultation postpartum amenorrhea
P_{PA}	pulmonary artery pressure
PPB	positive pressure breathing prepatellar bursitis
PPBS	postprandial blood sugar
PPC	pooled platelet concentrate progressive patient care pseudopurulent conjunctivitis
PP & C	prefabricated post and core (dentistry)
PPD	percussion and postural drainage progressive pulmonary dystrophy purified protein derivative (procedure/tuberculin skin test)
PPF	palmoplantar fibromatosis plasma protein fraction postprandial fullness
PPG	photoplethysmograph postpartum galactorrhea

PPH	postpartum hemorrhage prepubertal panhypopituitarism primary pulmonary hypertension
PPHP	pseudo-pseudohypoparathyroidism
Ppl	pleural pressure
PPLO	pleuropneumonia-like organism
PPM	permanent pacemaker
ppm	parts per million
PPMA	progressive postpoliomyelitis atrophy
PPO	participating providers organization
PPP	palmoplantar pustulosis pentose phosphate pathway platelet-poor plasma postpartum psychosis
PPPPP	pain, pallor, pulse-loss, paresthesia, paralysis
PPR	per patient's request
PPRF	pontine paramedian reticular formation
PPS	postpartum sterilization protein plasma substitute
PPT	partial prothrombin time pneumonia prevention therapy (AIDS)
ppt	precipitate
PPTL	postpartum tubal ligation

PPV	positive pressure ventilation (respiratory therapy)
PQ	permeability quotient
PR	panic reaction partial remission peer review perfusion rate peripheral resistance pulmonary rehabilitation pulmonic regurgitation pulse rate
Pr	presbyopia (eye examination)
pr	pair per rectum
P & R	pelvic and rectal (examination) pulse and respiration
PRA	plasma renin activity (laboratory/endocrinology)
prac	practice
PRAS	prereduced (and) anaerobically sterilized
PRAT	platelet radioactive antiglobulin test
PRBC	packed red blood cells (blood transfusion)
PRBV	placental residual blood volume
PRC	plasma renin concentration
PRCA	primary red cell aplasia
PRD	postradiation dysplasia

PRDF	progressive recurrent dermatofibrosarcoma
PRE	progressive resistive exercises (physical therapy)
preauth	insurance preauthorization
pref	preference
preg	pregnant
pregang	preganglionic
prelim	preliminary
premed	premedication
premie	premature infant
prenat	prenatal
preop	preoperative
prep	prepare
press	pressure
prev	prevent previous
PRF	progressive renal failure prolactin releasing factor
PRG	phleborrheogram (hematology)
primip	primipara (woman bearing first child)
princ	principal principle

PRIST	paper radioimmunosorbent test
priv	private privilege
PRK	photorefractive keratectomy
PRL	prolactin
PRN	postrotatory nystagmus
prn	whenever necessary (Latin: *pro re nata*)
prob	probable
proc	procedure proceeding process
procto	proctoscopy
prod	product
prof	profession
proj	project
PROM	premature rupture of membranes
prom	prominent
pron	pronation
proph	prophylactic
prost	prostate
prosth	prosthesis
prot	protein

Pro-X	prothrombin time
prox	proximal
PRP	platelet-rich plasma (transfusion) pressure-rate product
PRRE	pupils round, regular, equal (eye examination)
PRT	photoradiation therapy
PRU	peripheral resistance unit
PS	performance status (rehabilitation) periodic syndrome physical status plastic surgery pleural space pulmonary stenosis pyloric stenosis
P/S	polyunsaturated to saturated fat ratio
P & S	paracentesis and suction
PSA	prostate-specific antigen
PSAGN	poststreptococcal acute glomerulonephritis
PSAT	prostate-specific antigen test
PSBO	partial small bowel obstruction
PSC	posterior subcapsular cataract primary sclerosing cholangitis pulse synchronized contractions
PSD	posterior sagittal diameter presenile dementia

PSE	portal systemic encephalopathy
PSF	posterior spinal function prestress fracture
PSG	pilot study group presenile gangrene presystolic gallop
pSG	peak systolic gradient
PSGN	poststreptococcal glomerulonephritis
PSH	past social history postspinal headache
PSI	posterior sagittal index
psi	pounds per square inch
PSIS	posterior superior iliac spine
PSL	potassium, sodium chloride, sodium lactate
PSM	presystolic murmur
PSMA	progressive spinal muscular atrophy
PSMF	protein-sparing modified fast
PSO	progressive supranuclear ophthalmoplegia
PSP	phenolsulfonphthalein (kidney function test) postsynaptic potential progressive supranuclear palsy
PSR	periodontal screening and recording problem status report

PSRBOW	premature spontaneous rupture of bag of waters
PSRO	Professional Standard Review Organization
PSS	partial striatal sclerosis physiological saline solution progressive systemic sclerosis
PST	pancreatic suppression test paroxysmal supraventricular tachycardia penicillin, streptomycin, tetracycline presenile tremor
PSU	postsurgical unit
PSV	pressure support ventilation
PSVER	pattern-shift visual evoked response
PSVT	paroxysmal supraventricular tachycardia
PSW	psychiatric social worker
PSY	psychiatry
PT	parathyroid paroxysmal tachycardia physical therapy physical training posterior tibial (pulse) prothrombin time pseudotumor pyramidal tract
P & T	permanent and total (disability)
Pt	platinum

pt	part patient pint point
PTA	parathyroid thymic aplasia percutaneous transluminal angioplasty persistent truncus arteriosus plasma thromboplastin antecedent (Factor X) posttraumatic amnesia pretreatment anxiety prior to admission (arrival) prothrombin activity
PTAG	target-attaching globulin precursor
p'tase	phosphatase (laboratory/chemistry)
PTAV	percutaneous transluminal aortic valvuloplasty
PTB	patella tendon bearing (cast) prior to birth
PTBD	percutaneous transhepatic biliary drainage
PTC	percutaneous transhepatic cholangiography plasma thromboplastin component (Factor IX) prothrombin complex
PTCA	percutaneous transluminal coronary angioplasty
PTD	permanent and total disability prior to discharge

PTE	parathyroid extract pretibial edema proximal tibial epiphysis pulmonary thromboembolism
PTED	pulmonary thromboembolic disease
PTF	parathyroid fever plasma thromboplastin factor posttransfusion fever
PTH	pathology parathyroid hormone posttransfusion hepatitis
PTHS	parathyroid hormone secretion (rate)
PTI	persistent tolerant infection
PTK	posttraumatic keratitis
PTL	preterm labor
PTLD	posttransplant lymphoproliferative disease prescribed tumor lethal dose
PTM	posttransfusion mononucleosis
Ptm	transmural pressure
PTMDF	pupils, tension, media, disc, fundus
PTP	periodic thyrotoxic paralysis posterial tibial pulse
Ptp	transpulmonary pressure
PTR	peripheral total resistance
P_{Tr}	inspiratory triggering pressure

PTS	permanent threshold shift prior to surgery
PTSD	posttraumatic stress disorder
PTT	partial thromboplastin time patellar tendon transfer pulmonary transit time
PTU	propylthiouracil
PtVP	portal venous pressure
PTX	parathyroidectomy pneumothorax
PU	passed urine peptic ulcer pregnancy urine
PUA	plasma uric acid
PUB	percutaneous umbilical blood (sampling)
PUC	pediatric urine collector
PUD	peptic ulcer disease
PuD	pulmonary disease
PUE	pyrexia (fever) of unknown etiology
PUFA	polyunsaturated fatty acid
PUH	pregnancy urine hormone
PUL	percutaneous ultrasonic lithotripsy
pulm	pulmonary

PUN	plasma urea nitrogen
PUO	pyrexia (fever) of unknown origin
PUPP	pruritic urticarial papillary plaques (obstetrics)
PUVA	psoralen and ultraviolet A (treatment for psoriasis)
PUVD	pulsed ultrasonic (blood) velocity detector
PUW	pickup walker
PV	paraventricular peripheral vascular peripheral vein picornavirus plasma volume polycythemia vera portal vein postvoiding pulmonary vein
P & V	pyloroplasty and vagotomy (operation/stomach)
PVA	polyvinyl alcohol
PVB	premature ventricular beat
PVC	polyvinyl chloride postvoiding cystogram premature ventricular contraction pulmonary venous congestion
$PVCO_2$	partial pressure of venous carbon dioxide
PVD	percussion, vibration, drainage peripheral vascular disease

PVD *(cont)*	posterior vitreous detachment (eye) premature ventricular depolarization pulmonary vascular disease
PVE	premature ventricular extrasystole prosthetic valve endocarditis
PvE	pelvic examination
PVEM	postvaccinal encephalomyelitis
PVEP	pattern visual evoked potential (neurology)
PVF	peripheral visual field portal venous flow primary ventricular fibrillation
PVH	perivascular hemorrhage
PVI	peripheral vascular insufficiency
PVM	proteins, vitamins, minerals
PVO_2	partial pressure of venous oxygen
PVOD	peripheral vascular occlusive disease pulmonary venous obstructive disease
PVP	peripheral venous pressure
PVR	peripheral vascular resistance pulmonary vascular resistance pulse-volume recording
PVS	percussion, vibration, suction persistent vegetative state premature ventricular systole preventricular stenosis pulmonic valve stenosis

PVT	paroxysmal ventricular tachycardia portal vein thrombosis pressure, volume, temperature
PW	plantar wart posterior wall
Pw	progesterone withdrawal
PWA	person with AIDS
PWARC	person with AIDS-related complex
PWB	partial weight-bearing
PWBC	peripheral white blood cells
PWC	physical work capacity
PWH	progressive weakness and hypotonia
PWI	posterior wall infarct
PWLV	posterior wall of left ventricle
PWOS	postworkout syncope
PWP	pulmonary wedge pressure
PWS	port wine stain
PX	pancreatectomy physical examination
Px	prognosis
PXE	pseudoxanthoma elasticum
PXM	projection x-ray microscope

p/y	pack years (cigarette smoking)
PYM	psychosomatic medicine
PZI	protamine zinc insulin
PZP	pregnancy zone protein

Q

Q	cardiac output coulombs (electrical unit) glutamine quantity quinidine quotient volume of blood flow
$\dot{Q}$	rate of blood flow
q	each every (Latin: *quaque*)
QA	qualitative assessment quality assurance Quatrefage angle (orthopedics)
qam	every morning
QAP	quality assurance program quinine, atabrine, plasmoquine
QAR	quantitative autoradiogram
Q_B	total body clearance
Qc	pulmonary capillary blood flow (perfusion)
QCA	quantitative coronary angiogram
Qco_2	microliters of carbon dioxide given off per milligram of tissue per hour
QCT	quantitative computerized tomography
qd	every day (Latin: *quaque die*)
q2d	every second day

QE	Queyrat's erythroplasia (dermatology)
QEE	quadriceps extension exercise
qh	every hour
q2h	every two hours
qhs	at bedtime
QI	Quetelex Index (weight-to-height ratio)
qid	four times a day (Latin: *quater in die*)
QJ	quadriceps jerk
QM	quinacrine mustard
QMT	quantitative muscle testing
QNS	quantity not sufficient (on laboratory reports)
QO_2	oxygen consumption
qO_2	oxygen quotient
$Q^{\circ}O_2$	oxygen consumption rate (microliters per milligram per hour)
qod	every other day
qoh	every other hour
QOL	quality of life
qon	every other night
QP	quadrant pain (gastroenterology)

Qp	pulmonary blood flow
QPC	quality of patient care
Q_{PC}	pulmonary capillary blood flow
QPD	qualitative platelet defect
QPEEG	qualitative pharmacoelectroencephalogram
qpm	every night
QP/QS	ratio of pulmonary to systemic circulation
qq	each
QRN	quality review nurse
QS	every shift (nursing)
qs	as much as will suffice (Latin: *quantum sufficit*) sufficient quantity (Latin: *quantum satis*) (prescriptions)
QS2	total electromechanical systole
qs ad	to a sufficient quantity (prescriptions)
Qs/Qt	intrapulmonary shunt ratio
QSS	quantitative sacroiliac scintigraphy
QT	Quick's test (obstetrics/hematology)
qt	quart
qty	quantity
quad	quadriplegic

qual qualitative

quant quantitative

QUICHA quantitative inhalation challenge apparatus

qv as much as you wish (Latin: *quantum vis*)

R

R	radioactive range rate reaction rectal (temperature) regression regular resistance respirations rhythm
Ⓡ	recall right
r	radius roentgen (x-ray measurement)
R-	Rinne's test negative (hearing test)
R+	Rinne's test positive (hearing test)
RA	refractory anemia renal artery repeat action residual air rheumatoid agglutinins rheumatoid arthritis right arm right atrial right auricle room air
R_A	airway resistance (pulmonary function test)
Ra	radium (nuclear medicine)
RAA	renin-angiotensin-aldosterone (system) right atrial abnormality

RA-ABG	room air arterial blood gases
RAB	rice, applesauce, banana (diet)
RAC	retinal arterial collapse right atrial catheter
RAD	radiation absorbed dose radiology reactive airways disease restricted activity day right axis deviation (ECG)
rad	radial radical
RADISH	rheumatoid arthritis diffuse idiopathic skeletal hyperostosis
RAE	right atrial enlargement
RAF	rheumatoid arthritis factor (laboratory/serology)
RAH	right anterior hemiblock right atrial hypertrophy
RAI	radioactive iodine (nuclear medicine) Respite Assessment Inventory right atrial involvement
RAIU	radioactive iodine uptake (nuclear medicine)
RALS	remote afterloading system
RALT	routine admission laboratory tests
RAO	right anterior oblique

RAP	renal arterial pressure right atrial pressure
RAPC	rheumatoid arthritis-pneumoconiosis
RAR	right arm recumbent
RAST	radioallergosorbent test (allergy) right anterior superior thorax
RAT	renal artery thrombosis repeat action tablet rheumatoid arthritis test right anterior thigh (injection site)
RATx	radiation therapy
RB	right bronchus right buttock (injection site)
rb	rebreathing
R & B	right and below
RBA	relative binding activity rescue breathing apparatus right brachial artery
RBB	right breast biopsy
RBBB	right bundle branch block (ECG)
RBC	red blood cell
RBCC	red blood cell cast
RBCD	right border of cardiac dullness
RBC/hpf	red blood cells per high power field

RBCM	red blood cell mass
RBCV	red blood cell volume (laboratory/hematology)
RBD	regular blood donor
RBF	renal blood flow
RBKA	right below-knee amputation
RBN	retrobulbar neuritis
RBOW	rupture of bag of waters (obstetrics)
RBP	resting blood pressure retinol binding protein
RBS	random blood smear
RC	respirations ceased respite care retention catheter retrograde cystogram
R/C	reclining chair
RCA	radionuclide cerebral angiogram red cell aplasia right coronary artery
rCBF	regional cerebral blood flow
RCC	rape crisis center red cell count renal cell carcinoma root canal completed (dentistry)
RCCA	right common carotid artery

RCD	relative (area of) cardiac dullness retinal cystoid degeneration
RCF	residential care facility
RCG	radiocardiogram
RCI	red cell indices
RCL	right coronary lesion
RCM	radiographic contrast media red cell mass right costal margin
RCP	riboflavin carrier protein
RCR	respiratory control ratio
RCS	repeat cesarean section reticulum cell sarcoma
RCT	random clinical trial red cell toxin root canal treatment (dentistry)
RCU	respiratory care unit
RCV	red cell volume (laboratory/hematology)
RD	Raynaud's disease Registered Dietitian renal disease respiratory disease retina detachment right deltoid (injection site) rubber dam (dentistry) ruptured disc

RDA	recommended dietary allowance right dorsoanterior
RDDA	recommended daily dietary allowance
RDE	receptor-destroying enzyme
RDFT	ratio of decayed to filled teeth
RDI	rupture delivery interval (obstetrics)
RDS	respiratory distress syndrome
RDT	regular dialysis treatment
RDVT	recurrent deep vein thrombosis
RE	rectal examination regional enteritis resting energy reticuloendothelium right extremity right eye
$\mathbf{R_E}$	respiratory exchange
REA	radioenzymatic assay
rec	record recurrent
RECA	right external carotid artery
RECG	radioelectrocardiogram
recip	recipient
recond	reconditioning

reconstr reconstruction

rect rectal
rectum

recur recurrence

REEG radioelectroencephalogram

REF renal erythropoietic factor

ref reference

REG radioencephalogram

reg region
registered
regular

regen regenerate

rehab rehabilitation

rel relation
relative

REM rapid eye movement (dream sleep)

REN reproductive endocrinology

ReoV reovirus

rep let it be repeated (Latin: *repetatur*) (prescriptions)
report

RER renal excretion rate
respiratory exchange ratio
rough endoplasmic reticulum

RES	reticuloendothelial system
res	research reserve resident
resp	respective respiration responsible
ret	retired
retic ct	reticulocyte count
retics	reticulocytes (laboratory/hematology)
RetV	retrovirus
rev	review revision
REx	resistive exercise
RF	receptive field (ophthalmology) relapsing fever renal failure respiratory failure reticular formation rheumatic fever rheumatoid factor
RFA	right femoral artery right forearm right frontoanterior (fetal position)
RFB	retained foreign body
RFD	rice-fruit diet
RFFIT	rapid fluorescent focus inhibition test

RFI request for information

RFLP restriction fragment length polymorphism (forensic blood test)

RFOL results to follow

RFP right frontoposterior (fetal position)

RFR refraction

RFS renal function studies

RFT right frontotransverse (fetal position)

RFV right femoral vein

RFX reflex

RG remotivation group (psychotherapy)
retrograde
right gluteus (injection site)

RGE relative gas expansion

RGP retrograde pyelogram

RGU renal glycosuria

RH reactive hyperemia
releasing hormone
right hand
room humidifier

Rh+, Rh- Rhesus positive, Rhesus negative (blood) (laboratory, blood bank)

RhA rheumatoid agglutinins (laboratory/serology)

RHB	right heart bypass
RHC	respirations have ceased reticulohistiocytoma
RHCF	residential health care facility
RHD	relative hepatic dullness renal hypertensive disease rheumatic heart disease
rheum	rheumatic
RhEx	rhythmic exercise
RHF	right heart failure
Rhf	Rhesus factor (laboratory/blood bank)
RHG	relative hemoglobin
RHH	right homonymous hemianopsia
RHI	rhinology
RHL	right hepatic lobe
rhm	roentgens per hour (at one) meter (radiation therapy)
RHOB	raise head of bed
RHP	right hemiparesis right hemiplegia
RHR	resting heart rate
RHT	right hypertropia (ophthalmology)
RHU	rheumatology

RhV	rhinovirus
RI	radiation intensity refractive index (eye examination) regional ileitis respiratory illness
RIA	radioimmunoassay (laboratory method)
RIC	right iliac crest right internal capsule right internal carotid
RICE	rest, ice, compression, elevation
RICS	right intercostal space
RICU	respiratory intensive care unit
RID	radial immunodiffusion
RIF	right iliac fossa (injection site) right internal fixation (orthopedics)
RIFA	radioiodinated fatty acid
RIG	rabies immune globulin
RIH	right inguinal hernia
RIHSA	radioiodinated human serum albumin
RIMA	right internal mammary anastomosis
RIND	reversible ischemic neurologic defect
RIP	radioisotopic pathology rapid infusion pump

RIPA radioimmunoprecipitin assay (HIV antibody test)

RIR right inferior rectus (muscle)

RISA radioactive iodinated serum albumin (nuclear medicine)

RIST radioimmunosorbent test (laboratory method)

RIU radioactive iodine uptake (nuclear medicine)

RIV right innominate vein

RIVS ruptured interventricular septum

RK radial keratotomy (operation/ophthalmology)
right kidney

RKY roentgen kymography

RL Record Librarian
right lateral
right leg
right lung
Ringer's lactate

R→L right to left

R_L respiratory resistance

RLB Rickettsia-like bodies

RLBCD right lower border of cardiac dullness

RLC residual lung capacity (pulmonary function test)

RLD	related living (organ) donor right lateral decubitus (position) ruptured lumbar disc
RLE	right lower extremity
RLF	retained lung fluid retrolental fibroplasia
RLL	right lower lobe (lung)
rll	right lower (eye)lid
RLN	regional lymph nodes
RLQ	right lower quadrant (abdomen)
RLR	right lateral rectus (eye muscle)
RLS	restless leg syndrome (sleep disorder) rheumatoid lung silicosis right-to-left shunt Ringer's lactate solution
RLSB	right lower sternal border
RLT	right lateral thigh (injection site)
RM	radical mastectomy (operation/breast) respiratory movement
Rm	remission (oncology)
RMA	right mentoanterior (fetal position)
RMB	right mainstem bronchus
RMCA	right main coronary artery
RMCL	right midclavicular line

RMD	rapid movement disorder (neurology)
RML	right mediolateral (episiotomy) (operation/obstetrics) right middle lobe (lung)
RMP	resting membrane potential right mentoposterior (fetal position)
RMR	resting metabolic rate right medial rectus (eye muscle)
RMS	respiratory muscle strength rhabdomyosarcoma
RMSF	Rocky Mountain spotted fever
RMT	right mentotransverse (fetal position)
RMV	respiratory minute volume (pulmonary function test)
RN	radionuclide Registered Nurse
Rn	radon (radiation measurement)
RNA	radionuclide angiography Registered Nurse Anesthetist ribonucleic acid
RNase	ribonuclease
RNBA	refractory normoblastic anemia
RND	radical neck dissection
RNP	ribonucleoprotein
RNS	reference normal serum

RNV	radionuclide venography
RO	radiation oncology reality orientation (psychiatry) reverse osmosis routine order
R/O	rule out
ROA	right occiput anterior (fetal position)
ROAD	reversible obstructive airway disease
ROD	renal osteodystrophy
ROI	region of interest (radiology)
ROM	range-of-motion rupture of membranes (obstetrics)
ROP	retinopathy of prematurity right occiput posterior (fetal position)
ROS	radiopaque swallow (diagnostic procedure) review of systems
ROSC	restoration of spontaneous circulation
ROT	remedial occupational therapy right occiput transverse (fetal position)
rot	rotate
rout	routine
RP	radial pulse Raynaud's phenomenon referring physician refractory period Registered Pharmacist

RP *(cont)* — relative potency
renal perfusion
resting potential
retinitis pigmentosa

R_P — pulmonary resistance (pulmonary function test)

RPA — radial photon absorptiometry
retroperitoneal adenitis
reverse passive anaphylaxis (allergy)
right pulmonary artery

RP & C — root planing and curettage (dentistry)

RPD — removable partial denture

RPF — Reiter protein (complement) fixation test (laboratory/serology)
relaxed pelvic floor
renal plasma flow

RPGN — rapidly progressive glomerulonephritis

RPH — retroperitoneal hemorrhage

RPHA — reverse passive hemagglutination

RPI — reticulocyte production index

RPICA — right posterior internal carotid artery

RPLND — retroperitoneal lymph node dissection

rpm — revolutions per minute

RPN — renal papillary necrosis

RPO — right posterior oblique (fetal position)

RPP	retinal periphlebitis retropubic prostatectomy (operation/urology)
RPR	rapid plasma reagin (test) (laboratory/serology)
RPS	renal pressor substance review per screen (radiology)
rps	revolutions per second
RPT	Registered Physical Therapist
rpt	repeat
rptd	ruptured
RPU	retropubic urethropexy
RPV	right pulmonary vein
RPx	revised prognosis
RQ	respiratory quotient
RR	radiation response recovery room regular respirations relative risk respiratory rate
R & R	rate and rhythm (heart) rest and relaxation
RRA	radioreceptor assay Registered Record Administrator
RRC	routine respiratory care

RRE	round, regular, equal (eye examination)
rRNA	ribosomal ribonucleic acid
RRP	relative refractory period (heart)
RRR	regular rate and rhythm (orthopedics)
RRRN	round, regular, react normally (pupils)
RRT	Registered Respiratory Therapist
RRV	rhesus rotavirus vaccine
RRx	radiation treatment
RS	rectal suppository (prescriptions) reinforcing stimulus review of symptoms Reye's syndrome rheumatoid spondylitis rhythm strip (electrocardiogram) right side Ringer's solution
R/S	reschedule
RSA	right sacroanterior right subclavian artery
RSB	right sternal border
RSBA	refractory sideroblastic anemia
RSC	reversible sickled cells
RScA	right scapuloanterior (fetal position)
RScP	right scapuloposterior (fetal position)

RSD	relative standard deviation
RSDS	reflex sympathetic dystrophy syndrome
RSIVP	rapid sequence intravenous pyelogram (x-ray/kidneys)
RSL	right sacrolateral (fetal position)
RSO	right-salpingo-oophorectomy (operation/gynecology)
RSP	rapid steady progression (prognosis) rhinoseptoplasty right sacroposterior (fetal position)
RSR	regular sinus rhythm (heart) relative survival rate (oncology)
RSS	right subscapular skinfold (thickness)
RST	radiosensitivity test rapid surfactant test reagin screen test right sacrotransverse (fetal position)
RSV	respiratory syncytial virus right subclavian vein
RSW	right-sided weakness (neurology)
RT	radiotherapy reaction time recreational therapy renal transplant respiratory therapy reverse transcriptase right thigh room temperature

R_T	total pulmonary resistance
rt	right
r/t	related to
RTA	renal tubular acidosis routine tests administered
RTC	return to clinic round the clock
RTF	residential treatment facility respiratory tract fluid
RTI	respiratory tract infection
Rti	tissue resistance
RTKP	radiothermokeratoplasty
RTL	reactive to light
rt lat	right lateral
RTN	renal tubular necrosis return routine tests negative
RTO	return to office
RTS	real-time scan (radiology)
RT_3U	resin triiodothyronine uptake (laboratory/endocrinology)
RTUS	real-time ultrasonography
RTx	radiation therapy

RU	radioactive uptake rectourethral residual urine resin uptake retrograde urogram right upper roentgen unit (radiation therapy)
RUA	right upper arm routine urinalysis
RUDS	random urine drug screen
RUE	right upper extremity
RUG	retrograde urethrogram
RUL	right upper lobe (lung)
rul	right upper (eye)lid
RUO	right ureteral orifice
rupt	rupture
RUQ	right upper quadrant
RUR	resin uptake ratio
RURTI	recurrent upper respiratory tract infection
RUSB	right upper sternal border
RV	residual volume (pulmonary function test) return visit right ventricle rotavirus rubella vaccine
RVA	rabies vaccine absorbed

RVA *(cont)*	reduced visual acuity renal vascular resistance right ventricular abnormality
RVD	relative vertebral density right ventricular dimension
RVDO	right ventricular diastolic overload
RVE	reduced ventilatory effort right ventricular enlargement
RVEDP	right ventricular end-diastolic pressure
RVET	right ventricular ejection time
RVF	right ventricular function
RVFP	right ventricular filling pressure
RVG	radionuclide ventriculography (procedure/cardiology)
RVH	renovascular hypertension right ventricular hypertrophy
RVID	right ventricular internal dimension
RVIDP	right ventricular initial diastolic pressure
RVO	relaxed vaginal outlet retinal vein occlusion right ventricular outflow
RVP	right ventricular pressure
RVR	renal vascular resistance renal vein renin

RVSW right ventricular stroke work

RVT renal vein thrombosis

RV/TLC residual volume per total lung compliance (pulmonary function test)

RVV rubella virus vaccine

Rx drugs
medication
prescription
take (Latin: *recipe*)
therapy
treatment

Rxn reaction

S

S	sacral (vertebrae) saline saturation section single (marital status) soft (diet) soluble son stimulus streptomycin suction surgery
S_1—S_4	heart sounds (first through fourth)
S1—S5	sacral vertebrae (1 through 5)
s	seconds sign
$\bar{s}$	without (Latin: *sine*)
SA	salicylic acid semen analysis serum albumin short-acting sinoatrial (node) sinus arrest sinus arrhythmia Stokes-Adams (attacks) suicide awareness surface area sustained action (drugs)
S/A	sugar and acetone (laboratory/urinalysis)
SAARD	slow-acting antirheumatic drug

SAB	subarachnoid block
SAb	spontaneous abortion
SABP	spontaneous acute bacterial peritonitis
SAC	short arm cast shoulder adhesive capsulitis
SACD	subacute combined degeneration
SACE	serum angiotensin-converting enzyme
SACH	solid ankle, cushion heel (prosthesis)
SACT	sinoatrial conduction time
SAD	seasonal affective disorder small airway disease
SADA	sugar, acetone, diacetic acid (test)
SADS	Self-Assessment Depression Scale sudden arrhythmic death syndrome
SAECG	signal-averaged electrocardiogram
SAED	selected area electron diffraction
SAFA	soluble antigen fluorescent antibody (test)
SAFE	stationary attachment, flexible endoskeleton
SAH	subarachnoid hemorrhage systemic arterial hypertension
SAI	short-acting insulin

SAIDS sexually acquired immuno-deficiency syndrome

SAIDs steroidal anti-inflammatory drugs

Sal Salmonella

sal salicylate

SAM scanning acoustic microscope
self-administered medication
systolic anterior motion

SAN sinoatrial node

SANC short arm navicular cast

sanit sanitary

SAO subclavian artery occlusion

SAO_2 arterial blood oxygen saturation

SAP serum alkaline phosphatase
service assessment program
systemic arterial pressure

SAPMS short arm posterior molded splint

SAQ short arc quadriceps (exercise)

SART sinoatrial recovery time

SAS short arm splint
signs and symptoms
sleep apnea syndrome
sterile aqueous suspension
subarachnoid space
supravalvular aortic stenosis

SASD	secundum atrial septal defect
SaSE	saline solution enema
sat	saturated
SATL	surgical Achilles tendon lengthening
SATS	Streptococcus A toxic shock
sat sol	saturated solution (prescriptions)
SAVD	spontaneous assisted vaginal delivery
SB	scleral buckling (eye) serum bilirubin single breath sinus bradycardia small bowel spina bifida sponge bath Stanford-Binet (intelligence test) sternal border stillborn suction biopsy
Sb	strabismus (eye examination)
SBA	sideroblastic anemia stand-by assistance (emergency medicine) subarachnoid block anesthesia
SBC	special back care strict bed confinement
SBD	straight bag drainage (urology)
SBE	self breast examination shortness of breath on exertion subacute bacterial endocarditis

SBF	splanchnic blood flow
SBFT	small bowel follow-through (x-ray)
SBGM	self blood glucose monitoring
SBI	systemic bacterial infection
SBJ	skin, bones, joints
SBMPL	simultaneous binaural midplane localization
SBN_2	single-breath nitrogen (test)
SBO	small bowel obstruction spina bifida occulta
SBP	spontaneous bacterial peritonitis steroid-binding plasma systolic blood pressure
SBR	strict bed rest
SBS	shaken baby syndrome short bowel syndrome sick building syndrome (environmental medicine)
SBSM	self blood sugar monitoring
SBW	seat belts worn (accident reports)
SC	sacrococcygeal scleral cautery (eye) self care service-connected (disability) sickle cell (anemia) skin conductance special care

SC *(cont)* — sternoclavicular (joint)
subclavian
subconjunctival
supportive care
supraclavicular

sc — without correction (eye examination)

SCA — selective coronary angiogram
sickle cell anemia
spinocerebellar ataxia
suspected child abuse

SCABG — single coronary artery bypass graft

SCAE — subcortical arteriosclerotic encephalopathy

SCAT — sheep cell agglutination test

SCB — strictly confined to bed

SCBA — self-contained breathing apparatus

SCC — short-course chemotherapy
spinal cord compression
squamous cell carcinoma
subcutaneous sarcoidosis

SCCL — small-cell carcinoma of the lung

SCD — service-connected disability
sickle cell disease
spinal cord disease
sudden cardiac death

SCE — subcutaneous emphysema

SCEMIA — self-contained enzymatic membrane immunoassay

SCFA	short-chain fatty acid
SCH	spinal cord hemangioma subconjunctival hemorrhage
SCHC	sickle cell-hemoglobin C disease
sched	schedule
SCHNC	squamous cell head and neck cancer
SCHT	subcutaneous histamine test
SCI	spinal cord injury
SCIDS	severe combined immune deficiency syndrome
SCIPP	sacrococcygeal to inferior pubic point
SCIV	subclavian intravenous (line)
SCK	serum creatine kinase
SCL	scleroderma soft contact lens
SCLC	small-cell lung carcinoma
SCLE	subacute cutaneous lupus erythematosus
SCM	sternocleidomastoid muscle
SCNS	subcutaneous nerve stimulation
scop	scopolamine
SCP	single-cell protein standard care plan

SCPK	serum creatine phosphokinase
SCR	skin conductance response spondylitic caudal radiculopathy
SCS	shaken child syndrome
SCT	sex chromatin test sickle cell trait staphylococcal clumping test
SCU	special care unit
SCUD	schizophrenia, chronic undifferentiated
SCV	smooth, capsulated, virulent (bacteria)
SCVB	subcutaneous vaginal block
SD	seizure disorder septal defect (heart) skin dose spontaneous delivery standard deviation sterile dressing sudden death
S & D	stomach and duodenum (x-ray)
SDA	shoulder disarticulation
SDAT	senile dementia of Alzheimer's type
SDB	self-destructive behavior subdeltoid bursitis
SDC	sleep disorders center
SDD	sterile dry dressing

SDH	subdural hematoma
SDI	state disability insurance
SDN	sporadic dysplastic nevi (dermatology)
SDP	single-donor platelets
SDS	same-day surgery sensory deprivation syndrome Shy-Drager syndrome
sds	sounds
SDU	short double upright (brace) step down unit
SE	saline enema sphenoethmoidal (suture) spin echo (radiology) staphylococcal enterotoxin standard error (laboratory) status epilepticus
^{75}Se	radioactive selenomethionine (nuclear medicine)
SEA	sheep erythrocyte agglutination (test)
SEC	serum electrolyte concentration sporadic erythrocytosis squamous epithelial cells
sect	section
SED	skin erythema dose
sed rate	sedimentation rate
SEEP	small end expiratory pressure

SEG	sonoencephalogram
segs	segmented neutrophils
SEL	spontaneous esophageal laceration
SEM	scanning electron microscope systolic ejection murmur
SEMI	subendocardial myocardial infarction
sem ves	seminal vesicles
SENA	sympathetic efferent nerve activity
sens	sensitivity (on culture reports)
SEP	sensory evoked potential Starr-Edwards prosthesis systolic ejection period
sep	separate
sept	septum
seq	sequence
SER	smooth endoplasmic reticulum somatosensory evoked response systolic ejection rate
Ser	serine
serv	service
SES	socioeconomic status
SET	skin endpoint titration surrogate embryo transfer (gynecology) systolic ejection time

SEV	Starr-Edwards (heart) valve
sev	several severe severed
SF	salt-free scarlet fever seminal fluid Streptococcus faecalis stress fracture symptom-free
sf	synovial fluid
S & F	soft and flat
SFA	saturated fatty acids superficial femoral artery
SFB	spinal fluid block
SFD	skin-to-film distance (radiology) small-for-dates (gynecology)
SFEMG	single-fiber electromyography
SFF	silver-fork fracture
SFOM	suppurative focal osteomyelitis
SFP	spinal fluid pressure
SFR	stroke with full recovery
SFS	serial focal seizures
SFT	skinfold thickness
SG	serum glucose

SG *(cont)*	skin graft specific gravity (urine)
SGA	senile genital atrophy small for gestational age
SGB	strawberry gallbladder
SGC	Swan-Ganz catheter
SGD	straight gravity drainage
SGE	significant glandular enlargement
SGF	skeletal growth factor
SGOT	serum glutamic oxaloacetic transaminase
SGP	soluble glycoprotein
SGPT	serum glutamic pyruvic transaminase
SGV & P	selective gastric vagotomy and pyloroplasty
SH	serum hepatitis sex hormone spinal headache surgical history
sh	short shoulder
S & H	speech and hearing
SHA	superheated aerosol
SHAA	serum hepatitis-associated antigen
SHB	scapulohumeral bursitis

SHb	sulfhemoglobin
SHBG	serum hemoglobin-blood glucose sex hormone-binding globulin
SHC	sinus histiocytosis
SHD	scapulohumeral dystrophy
SHEENT	skin, hair, eyes, ears, nose, throat
Shig	Shigella (laboratory/bacteriology)
SHN	spontaneous hemorrhagic necrosis
SHO	secondary hypertrophic osteoarthropathy
SHP	Schonlein-Henoch purpura
SHx	social history
SI	sacroiliac saline injection saturation index self-inflicted serum iron soluble insulin special intervention stress incontinence stroke index
Si	silicon
SIA	stress-induced anesthesia
SIADH	serum-inappropriate antidiuretic hormone
SIB	self-injurious behavior
sib	sibling

SICU	surgical intensive care unit
SIDS	sudden infant death syndrome
SIE	subacute infective endocarditis
SIg	serum immune globulin
sig	let it be labeled (Latin: *signetur*) significant
sigmo	sigmoidoscopy (procedure/intestinal)
SIJ	sacroiliac joint
SIMS	surgical indication monitoring system
SIMV	synchronized intermittent mandatory ventilation
SIP	sickness impact profile
SIRS	systemic inflammatory response syndrome
SIS	sterile injectable suspension
SISI	short increment sensitivity index
SIV	simian immunodeficiency virus
SIW	self-inflicted wound
SK	streptokinase
sk	skeletal
SKS	syphilitic knee synovitis
SKSD	streptokinase-streptodornase

SL sensation level
serotonin level
serum lipid
slit lamp (eye examination)
sound level
streptolysin
sublingual

sl slight
slow

SLA left sacroanterior (fetal position)
slide latex agglutination

SLB short leg brace

SLC short leg cast

SLD school-loss day

SLE systemic lupus erythematosus

SLEV St. Louis encephalitis virus

SLFIA substrate-linked fluorescent immunoassay

SLM spatial light modulator

SLMFD sterile low midforceps delivery

SLO streptolysin-O

SLP left sacroposterior (fetal position)

SLPMS short leg posterior molded splint

SLR straight leg raising

SLS short leg splint

SLT	sex-linked thrombocytopenia
sl/tr	slight trace (on laboratory reports)
SLWC	short leg walking cast
SM	self-medication self-monitoring simple mastectomy skim milk smooth muscle sphingomyelin spinal manipulation (osteopathy) streptomycin submucosal systolic mean (pressure) systolic murmur
sm	small
SMA	smooth muscle antibody spinal muscular atrophy superior mesenteric artery
SMA-6, -12	Sequential Multiple Analysis tests
SMAO	superior mesenteric artery occlusion
SMBG	self-monitored blood glucose
SMC	smooth muscle cell somatomedin C special mouth care
SMD	senile macular degeneration submanubrial dullness
SMI	supplementary medical insurance sustained maximal inspiration

SMO	slip made out (laboratory)
SMON	subacute myelooptic neuropathy
SMP	self-management program
SMPC	submucous palatal cleft
SMR	skeletal muscle relaxant (drug) somnolent metabolic rate standard mortality rate submucous resection (operation/nose)
SMS	serial motor seizures
SMT	stress management training
SMVT	sustained monomorphic ventricular tachycardia
SMX	sulfamethoxazole
SN	sinus node staff nurse standard nomenclature (records) student nurse subnormal suprasternal notch
S/N	sample to negative control ratio signal to noise ratio
SNAP	sensory nerve action potential
SNB	scalene node biopsy (operation/chest)
SNCV	sensory nerve conduction velocity
SND	sinus node disease

SNE	subacute necrotizing encephalomyopathy
SNF	skilled nursing facility
SNGFR	single nephron glomerular filtration rate
SNHL	sensorineural hearing loss
SNO	substantive negative outcome
SNOP	Standard Nomenclature of Pathology
SNP	sodium nitroprusside
SNRT	sinus node recovery time
SNS	sympathetic nervous system
SNV	systemic necrotizing vasculitis
SO	salpingo-oophorectomy second opinion sex offender significant other suicide observation superior oblique supraoptic
sO_2	blood oxygen saturation
SO_4	sulphate
SOA	supraorbital artery (neurological test)
SOAA	signed out against advice
SOAE	spontaneous otoacoustic emission
SOAP	subjective (data), objective (data), assessment, plan (medical records)

SOAPS	suction, oxygen, apparatus, pharmaceutics, saline (treatment procedure)
SOB	short of breath
SOBT	solution-oriented brief therapy (psychiatry)
SOC	standard of care
S&OC	signed and on chart
SOI	severity of illness
SOL	space-occupying lesion
sol	solution (prescriptions)
solv	dissolve (Latin: *solve*) (prescriptions) solvent
SOM	serous otitis media superior oblique muscle (eye)
SOMA	signed out against medical advice
SOMI	sternooccipital mandibular immobilization
SONP	solid organs not palpable
SOP	spinal osteophytosis standard operating procedure
SOPWAs	survivors of a person with AIDS
SOS	shortness of stature supplemental oxygen system
SOV	Sabin oral vaccine (poliomyelitis)
SP	sequential pulse

SP *(cont)*	speech pathology standard practice status positive suicide precaution suprapubic symphysis pubis systolic pressure
sp	space species specific spinal
S/P	sacrum to pubis (surgery) semi-private (room) status post (no change — as before)
SPA	salt-poor albumin (intravenous therapy) spondyloarthropathy suprapubic aspiration
SPAD	subcutaneous peritoneal access device
spans	spansules (prescriptions)
SPBI	serum protein-bound iodine
SPBT	suprapubic bladder tap
SPC	standard platelet count
SPCA	serum prothrombin conversion accelerator (Factor VII)
sp/cd	spinal cord
SPD	sociopathic personality disorder
SPE	serum protein electrolytes

spec	special specific specimen speculum
SPECT	single-photon-emission computed tomography
SPEP	serum protein electrophoresis
SPES	short psychiatric evaluation scale
SPF	skin protection factor
SPFI	solid-phase fluorescent immunoassay
sp/fl	spinal fluid
SPG	specific gravity
SPH	secondary pulmonary hemosiderosis suprarenal pseudohermaphroditism
Sph	sphingomyelin
sph	spherical
SPLATT	split anterior tibial transfer
SPO	status postoperative
spon	spontaneous
SPP	suprapubic prostatectomy
spp	species
SPPS	stable plasma protein solution
SPRIA	solid-phase radioimmunoassay

SPROM	spontaneous premature rupture of membranes
SPS	spastic pseudosclerosis systematic problem-solving (psychiatry)
SPT	skin prick test (allergy) suprapubic tube
SPU	short procedure unit
SPV	slow phase velocity
SPVR	systemic peripheral vascular resistance
SQ	subcutaneous (injection site)
sq	squamous (cell) square
SqCa	squamous cell carcinoma
SqEp	squamous epithelium
SQUID	superconducting quantum interference device
SR	sarcoplasmic reticulum secretion rate sedimentation rate side rails (bed) sinus rhythm (heart) skin resistance spontaneous remission stretch reflex sustained release (dosage) suture removal systems review (patient's history)
^{85}Sr	radioactive strontium (nuclear medicine)

SRBC sheep red blood cells

SRBOW spontaneous rupture of bag of waters

SRF skin reactive factor
somatotropin-releasing factor

SRFS split renal function study

SRH single radical hemolysis
spontaneously resolving hyperthyroidism

SRI severe renal insufficiency

SRM superior rectus muscle (eye)

SRMC single-room maternity care

SRN subretinal neovascularization

sRNA soluble ribonucleic acid

SR/NE sinus rhythm/no ectopy

SROM spontaneous rupture of membranes (obstetrics)

SRR surgical recovery room

SRS slow-reacting substance
splenorenal shunt

SRT sedimentation rate test
simple reaction time
speech reception threshold

SRU side rails up (bed)

SrU strontium unit

SS saline soak
saliva sample
salt substitute
saturated solution (prescriptions)
serum sickness
short stay (hospital)
siblings
side to side
skull series (radiology)
slip sent (laboratory)
smoking status
Social Security
social services
somatostatin
statistically significant
sterile solution
subaortic stenosis
substernal
supersaturated

S & S signs and symptoms
support and stimulation

$\overline{\text{ss}}$ one-half (Latin: *semissen*)
(medications orders/prescriptions)

SSA side-to-side anastomosis
skin-sensitizing antibody

SSC subcutaneous sarcoidosis

SSCA single shoulder contrast arthrography

SSCP single-strand conformation polymorphism

SSD source-to-skin distance (radiation)

SSE skin self-examination
soapsuds enema
systemic side effects

SSEP somatosensory evoked potential

SSI segmental sequential irradiation

SSKI saturated solution of potassium iodide

SSLE subacute sclerosing leukoencephalitis

SSLI serum sickness-like illness

SSM superficial spreading melanoma
suprasellar meningioma

SSMP spastic spinal monoplegia

SSO second surgical opinion

SSOC site-specific ovarian cancer

SSPE subacute sclerosing panencephalitis

SSR surgical supply room

SSRI selective serotonin reuptake inhibitor

SSS sick sinus syndrome
sterile saline soak
strong soap solution

SSSS staphylococcal scalded skin syndrome

SSU self-service unit

SSV simian sarcoma virus

SSX sulfisoxazole

ST serotonin
sinus tachycardia
skin tag

ST *(cont)*	speech therapist split thickness (graft) stress test surface tension survival time (oncology) symptomatic therapy
S/T	sulfamethoxazole and trimethoprim (antibacterial)
STA	spinothalamic ataxia superficial temporal artery
STAG	split thickness autogenous graft
staph	staphylococcus
stat	immediately (Latin: *statim*)
STB	silicotuberculosis
stb	stillborn
STC	soft tissue calcification stroke treatment center
STD	sexually transmitted disease short-term disability skin test dose skin-to-tumor distance (radiation) standard test dose
std	standard
STET	submaximal treadmill exercise test
stet	let it stand
STF	special tube feeding specialized treatment facility

STG	short-term goal (rehabilitation) split thickness graft
STH	soft tissue hematoma somatotropic (growth) hormone subtotal hysterectomy
STI	systolic time interval
stim	stimulus
STK	streptokinase
STLS	surface tension-lowering substance
STML	short-term memory loss
STP	sodium thiopental standard temperature and pressure
STR	stretcher
str	straight
strab	strabismus (eye examination)
strep	streptococcus
struc	structure
STS	serologic test for syphilis soft tissue swelling standard test for syphilis
STSD	secondary traumatic stress disorder
STSG	split thickness skin graft
STT	serial thrombin time

STU	skin test unit
SU	sensation unit stress ulcer
S & U	supine and upright
SUA	serum uric acid
subac	subacute
subcrep	subcrepitant (rales)
subling	sublingual (under tongue)
submand	submandibular
SUD	skin unit dose sudden unexplained death
SUDS	single unit delivery system sudden unexpected death syndrome
SUF	sequential ultrafiltration
suff	sufficient
SUID	sudden unexplained infant death
SUN	serum urea nitrogen
sup	superficial superior supination
supp	suppository suppurative
surf	surfactant

surg	surgery
SURT	sarcoidosis of upper respiratory tract
SUS	sustained urinary sediment
susp	suspension
SUX	succinylcholine
SV	simian virus sinus venosus snake venom stroke volume subclavian vein supraventricular
S/V	surface to volume ratio
SVAS	supravalvular aortic stenosis
SVB	saphenous vein bypass (graft)
SVC	selective venous catheterization slow vital capacity superior vena cava
SVCG	spatial vectorcardiogram
SVD	spontaneous vaginal delivery
SVE	sterile vaginal examination supraventricular ectopic (beat)
SVG	saphenous vein graft
SVI	small volume infusion stroke volume index
SVPB	supraventricular premature beat

SVPT	supraventricular paroxysmal tachycardia
SVR	slow vertex response supervoltage radiation supraventricular rhythm systemic vascular resistance
SVT	supraventricular tachycardia
SW	seriously wounded social worker stab wound stroke work
S & W	soap and water (enema)
SWD	shortwave diathermy
SWE	slow-wave encephalography
SWI	stroke work index surgical wound infection
SWIM	sperm-washing insemination method
SWR	serum Wassermann reaction
SWS	slow-wave sleep Sturge-Weber syndrome
SWU	septic workup
SX	surgeries
Sx	symptoms
S_x	signs
sx	suction

sym	symmetric
symp	sympathetic (nervous system)
syn	syndrome synovial (fluid) synovitis
sync	synchronous
syph	syphilis
syr	syrup (prescriptions)
sys	system
syst	systolic
Sz	schizophrenia seizure

T

T	tablespoonful temperature tension (pressure) thoracic topical (medication) total Treponema transverse tumor
t	teaspoonful three times (Latin: *ter*) time trace
T½	halflife
T_1, T_2	tricuspid heart sounds (first, second)
T1, T2	thoracic vertebrae (first, second)
T-1, T-2,...	stages of decreased intraocular tension
T+1, T+2	stages of increased intraocular tension
T_3	triiodothyronine
T_4	thyroxine
TA	temporary abstinence tension applantation (ophthalmology) therapeutic abortion toothache toxin-antitoxin tricuspid atresia truncus arteriosus
T(A)	temperature, axillary

T & A	tonsillectomy and adenoidectomy
TAA	thoracic aortic aneurysm total ankle arthroplasty tumor-associated antigen
tab	tablet
TABC	total aerobic bacteria count
TAC	terminal atrial contraction
TACE	tripara-anisylchloroethylene
tach	tachycardia
TAD	transverse abdominal diameter
TAE	transcatheter arterial embolization
TAF	traumatic aortocaval fistula tumor angiogenesis factor
TAG	target-attaching globulin thymine, adenine, guanine
TAH	total abdominal hysterectomy
TAL	tendo Achilles lengthening
TAM	tamoxifen toxin-antitoxin mixture treat arrhythmias medically
TAN	total ammonia nitrogen
TANI	total axial (lymph) node irradiation
TAO	thromboangiitis obliterans

TAPVD	total anomalous pulmonary venous drainage
TAR	total ankle replacement treatment authorization request
TARA	total articular replacement arthroplasty tumor-associated rejection antigen
TAS	thoracoabdominal stapler
TAT	tetanus antitoxin Thematic Apperception Test thromboplastin activation test
TATST	tetanus antitoxin skin test
TB	total base total body tracheobronchitis tubercle bacillus tuberculosis
TBA	thyroxine-binding albumin to be admitted (hospital)
TBB	transbronchial biopsy
TBC	thyroxine-binding coagulin
TBF	temporal bone fracture total body fat
TBG	thyroxin-binding globulin
TBH	total body hematocrit
TBI	total body irradiation traumatic brain injury

TBIL	total bilirubin
TBK	total body potassium
TBLC	term birth, live child
TBM	tuberculous meningitis
TBNA	treated but not admitted
TBP	thyroxine-binding protein
TBR	total bed rest
TBS	total body solute tubular bones stenosis
TBSA	temporal bone subperiosteal abscess total burn surface area
tbsp	tablespoonful
TBT	tolbutamine test tracheobronchial tree
TBV	total blood volume transluminal balloon valvuloplasty
TBW	total body water total body weight
TBZ	tetrabenazine (anesthetic adjuvant)
TC	tetracycline throat culture tissue culture total capacity (lung) total cholesterol total colonoscopy

TC *(cont)*	treatment completed tubocurarine
T & C	turn and cough type and crossmatch (laboratory/blood bank)
^{99m}Tc	radioactive technetium (nuclear medicine)
TCA	terminal cancer transluminal coronary angioplasty tricyclic antidepressant
TCABG	triple coronary artery bypass graft
TCAT	transmission computer-assisted tomography tricyclic antitussant
TCB	to call back
$TCCO_2$	transcutaneous carbon dioxide (monitor)
TC & DB	turn, cough and deep breathe
TCES	transcutaneous cranial electrical stimulation
TCF	total coronary flow
TCH	temporary contralateral hemiplegia total circulating hemoglobin traumatic cephalohydrocele
TCI	to come in (hospital) transient cerebral ischemia tricuspid insufficiency
TCID	tissue culture infective dose

TCIE	transient cerebral ischemic episode
TCM	tissue culture medium transcutaneous monitor
TCMI	T-cell-mediated immunity
TCNS	transcutaneous nerve stimulation
TCOM	transcutaneous oxygen monitor
$TCpO_2$	transcutaneous oxygen partial pressure
TCR	tricuspid regurgitation (cardiology)
TCT	thrombin clotting time tubocurarine test (diagnostic procedure)
TD	tardive dyskinesia thermal dysregulation thoracic duct threshold dose tic douloureux total disability toxic dose transverse diameter (of heart)
T_4D	thyroxine displacement (assay)
TD_{50}	median toxic dose
T/D	tetanus and diphtheria (toxoids) treatment discontinued
TDA	therapeutic drug assay
TDD	telecommunication device for the deaf thoracic duct drainage total digitalizing dose

TDE two-dimensional echocardiography

TDF tumor dose fractionation

TDK tardive dyskinesia

TDL thoracic duct lymphocytes

TDM therapeutic drug monitoring

TDN totally digestible nutrients

TDP transdermal patch

TDT tone decay test

TE tennis elbow
thromboembolism
tooth extracted
tracheoesophageal

T_E expiratory phase time

t_e effective half-life

T & E trial and error

TEA total elbow arthroplasty
total endoarterectomy

teasp teaspoonful

TEB transcutaneous endomyocardial biopsy

TeBG testosterone-binding globulin

TEC total eosinophil count

TED threshold erythema dose
thromboembolic disease

TEDS	thromboembolus deterrent stocking
TEE	thermal effect of exercise transesophageal echocardiogram
TEF	thermal effect of food tracheoesophageal fistula
TEG	thromboelastogram
TEM	transmission electron microscope triethylenemelamine (cancer chemotherapy)
temp	temperature temporal temporary
TEN	total enteral nutrition toxic epidermal necrolysis
TENS	transcutaneous electrical nerve stimulation
TEP	thromboendophlebectomy
TEPH	thromboembolic pulmonary hypertension
TER	total endoplasmic reticulum
term	terminal terminate
tert	tertiary
TET	treadmill exercise test
tet tox	tetanus toxoid (medication order)

TF	tactile fremitus tetralogy of Fallot to follow total flow transfer factor tube feeding
TFA	total fatty acids
TFB	trifascicular block (heart)
TFC	total food consumption
TFEV	timed forced expiratory volume
TF/P	tubular fluid-plasma ratio
TFR	total fertility rate
TFS	testicular feminization syndrome
TFT	thyroid function test
TG	tendon graft thyroglobulin toxic goiter triglycerides
TGA	transient global amnesia transposition of the great arteries
TGF	transformin growth factor
TGFA	triglyceride fatty acid
TGL	triglyceride level triglyceride lipase
TGN	trigeminal neuralgia (tic douloureux)

TGT	thromboplastin generation test
TGV	thoracic gas volume transposition of the great vessels
TH	tentorial herniation thyroid hormone (thyroxine) total hysterectomy
THA	total hip arthroplasty
Thal	thalassemia
THC	transhepatic cholangiography
TH & C	terpin hydrate and codeine
THE	transhepatic embolization
ther	therapy
therm	thermal thermometer
THF	tetrahydrofolate
Thg	thyroglobulin
TH_2O	titrated water
thor	thoracic
THR	target heart rate thyroid hormone receptor total hip replacement
ThRIA	thyroid radioisotope assay
throm	thrombosis

TI	thoracic index time interval tricuspid insufficiency
T_I	inspiratory phase time
TIA	transient ischemic attack
TIBC	total iron-binding capacity
TIC	trypsin inhibitory capacity
TID	titrated initial dose
tid	three times daily (Latin: *ter in die*)
TIE	transient ischemic episode
TIF	tumor-inducing factor
TIG	tetanus immune globulin
TIM	transthoracic intracardiac monitoring
TIN	tubulointerstitial nephropathy
tinct	tincture (prescriptions)
TIP	terbutaline infusion pump
TIPS	transjugular intrahepatic portosystemic shunt
TIR	terminal innervation ratio
TIRI	total immunoreactive insulin
TIS	tumor in situ
TIT	Treponema immobilization test

T_I/T_E	inspiratory-expiratory phase time ratio
titr	titrate (on prescriptions)
TIUV	total intrauterine volume
TJ	triceps jerk (neurologic examination)
tj	tendon jerk (orthopedics)
TJR	total joint replacement
TK	through the knee tourniquet
TKA	total knee arthroplasty
TKG	tokodynagraph
TKO	to keep open (intravenous therapy)
TKP	thermokeratoplasty
TKR	total knee replacement
TL	Team Leader temporal lobe time-limited total lipids tubal ligation
T/L	terminal latency (electromyogram)
TLA	transluminal angioplasty
TLAA	T-lymphocyte-associated antigen
TLC	tender loving care thin-layer chromatography

TLC *(cont)*	total lung capacity total lung compliance total lymphocyte count
TLD	transluminescent dosimeter tumor lethal dose
TLE	thin-layer electrophoresis
TLI	total lymphoid irradiation
TLmA	translumbar arteriogram
TLS	thoracolumbosacral (drain)
TLV	total lung volume
TM	temporomandibular (joint) tobramycin transmetatarsal (foot) transport mechanism tympanic membrane (ear)
Tm	maximum tubular clearance
TMA	transmetatarsal amputation
TMB	transient monocular blindness
TMC	transmural colitis (Crohn's)
TME	transmural enteritis
TMET	treadmill exercise test
Tm_G	maximum glucose reabsorptive capacity
TMI	threatened myocardial infarction transmural infarction

TMJ	temporomandibular joint
TMP	thallium myocardial perfusion (test) transmembrane pressure trimethoprim
Tm_{PAH}	maximum tubular excretory capacity for para-aminohippurate
TMS	thallium myocardial scintigraphy
TMT	tympanic membrane thermometer
TMTC	too many to count (laboratory)
TMV	tobacco mosaic virus
TMX	tamoxifen
TN	true negative
Tn	intraocular tension, normal
TND	term normal delivery transient neonatal diabetes
TNF	tumor necrosis factor
TNI	total nodal irradiation
T/NM	tumor with node metastasis
TNPM	transient neonatal pustular melanosis
TNTC	too numerous to count (laboratory)
TO	target organ tincture of opium tuboovarian

T(O)	temperature, oral (on temperature records)
T/O	telephone order
TOA	time of arrival (hospital) transposition of the aorta tuboovarian abscess
TOF	tetralogy of Fallot
TOGV	transposition of the great vessels
tomo	tomogram
TOP	termination of pregnancy
top	topical (medication orders/prescriptions)
TOPS	total ozone portable spectrometer
TOPV	trivalent oral poliomyelitis vaccine
TORCH	toxoplasmosis, rubella, cytomegalovirus and herpes simplex virus
TORP	total ossicular replacement prosthesis
TOVF	testing of visual fields
TOWER	testing, orientation, work, evaluation, rehabilitation
tox	toxic toxin
TP	temperature and pressure testosterone propionate therapeutic profile threshold potential thrombocytopenic purpura

TP *(cont)*	thrombophlebitis toilet paper total protein Treponema pallidum (syphilis) true positive tuberculin precipitation
TPA	third party administration tumor polypeptide antigen
tPA	tissue-plasminogen activator
TPB	transient posttraumatic blindness
TPBF	total pulmonary blood flow
TPBS	three-phase (radionuclide) bone scan
TPC	thromboplastic plasma component total patient care (nursing) transverse palmar crease (dermatology)
TPCF	Treponema pallidum complement fixation
TPCV	total packed cell volume
TPE	therapeutic plasma exchange
$\mathbf{T^{Pe}}$	expiratory pause time
TPG	transplacental gradient
TPH	thromboembolic pulmonary hypertension transient postictal hemianopsia transplacental hemorrhage
TPHA	Treponema pallidum hemagglutination
TPI	Treponema pallidum immobilization

T^Pi	inspiratory pause time
TPIA	Treponema pallidum immune adherence
TPM	temporary pacemaker
TPN	total parenteral nutrition
TP & P	time, place and person
TPR	temperature, pulse, respirations testosterone production rate total peripheral resistance total pulmonary resistance
TPT	total protein tuberculin typhoid-paratyphoid (vaccine)
TPTX	thyroid-parathyroidectomy
TPUR	transperineal urethral resection
TPVR	total peripheral vascular resistance
Tq	tourniquet
TR	therapeutic radiology total resistance true reading tricuspid regurgitation tubular resorption
T-R	test-retest
T(R)	temperature, rectal
tr	tincture trace traction tremor

TRA	tumor rejection antigen
trach	tracheotomy
trach asp	tracheal aspiration
trans	transverse
trans/d	transverse diameter
transm	transmission
transpl	transplant (transplantation)
TRBF	total renal blood flow (test)
TRC	total renin concentration
Trch	Trichophyton
TRCV	total red cell volume
TRD	tongue retaining device
TRE	traumatic retinal edema
Trend	Trendelenburg (position)
Trep	Treponema (on laboratory reports)
TRF	thyrotropin releasing factor
TRH	thyrotropin releasing hormone
T_3RIA	triiodothyronine radioimmunoassy
T_4RIA	thyroxine radioisotope assay
TRIC	trachoma inclusion conjunctivitis

trig triglycerides

TRM-SMX trimethoprim-sulfamethoxazole (antimicrobial)

tRNA transfer ribonucleic acid

TRP total refraction period (orthopedics)
tubular reabsorption of phosphate

Trp tryptophan

trt treatment

T_3RU triiodothyronine resin uptake

TRUS transrectal ultrasonography

Tryp Trypanosoma

TS test solution
thoracic surgery
total solids
Tourette syndrome
toxic shock
toxic substance
transverse section
tricuspid stenosis (heart)
trimethoprim-sulfamethoxazole (antimicrobial)
triple-strength

T/S thyroid-serum iodide ratio

TSA tissue-specific antigen
tumor-specific antigen

TSBB transtracheal selective bronchial brushing

TSD Tay-Sachs disease

TSE	testicular self-examination
T-sect	transverse (cross) section
T-set	tracheotomy set
TSF	triceps skinfold
TSG	tumor suppression gene
TSH	thyroid stimulating hormone
TSH-RF	thyroid stimulating hormone-releasing factor
TSI	thyroid-stimulating immunoglobulin
TSP	total serum protein
tsp	teaspoon
TSR	thyroid-serum ratio total shoulder replacement
tsr	transfer
TSS	toxic shock syndrome
TST	total sleep time treadmill stress test tumor skin test
TSTA	tumor-specific tissue antigen
T_3SU	triiodothyronine serum uptake
TT	tendon transfer tetanus toxoid therapeutic touch (nursing action)

TT *(cont)*	thrombin time thymol turbidity tibial torsion tilt table transit time (blood) transthoracic
TTA	total toe arthroplasty transtracheal aspiration
TTD	tissue tolerance doce (radiation)
TTH	thyrotropic hormone
TTI	tissue thromboplastin inhibition (test)
TTM	transtelephonic monitoring
TTN	transient tachypnea of the newborn
TTO	to take out
TTP	temporary transvenous pacemaker thrombotic thrombocytopenic purpura thyrotoxic paralysis
TTS	through the skin
TTT	tolbutamide tolerance test
TU	toxin unit transmission unit tuberculin unit
TUD	total urethral discharge
TUG	total urinary gonadotropin
T_3up	triiodothyronine uptake

T_4up	thyroxine uptake
TURB	transurethral resection of bladder
TURP	transurethral resection of prostate
tuss	cough (Latin: *tussis*)
TV	tidal volume (pulmonary function test) total volume Trichomonas vaginalis
tv	transvenous
TVC	timed vital capacity total volume capacity transvaginal cone triple voiding cystogram
TVCS	transverse vertical cross section
TVF	tactile vocal fremitis
TVG	transvalvular gradient
TVH	total vaginal hysterectomy
TVP	transvenous pacemaker transvesical prostatectomy tricuspid valve prolapse
TVR	tonic vibration reflex total vascular resistance tricuspid valve replacement
TVU	total volume urine
TVUS	transvaginal ultrasound

TW tap water
thin-walled
total (body) water

TWE tap water enema

Tx therapy
traction
transfusion
transplantation
treatment

T & X type and crossmatch

TXT treadmill exercise test

Ty type
typhoid

tymp tympanic (membrane)

Tyr tyrosine

U

U	units upper urology
u	units
UA	uric acid urinalysis uterine aspiration
UAC	umbilical artery catheter
UA/C	uric acid-creatinine ratio
UAD	upper airway disease uric acid dysmetabolism
UAN	uric acid nitrogen
UAO	upper airway obstruction
UAP	upper airway patency
UARS	upper airway resistance syndrome
UAS	uterine arteriosclerosis
UBB	unconjugated benign bilirubinemia
UBF	uterine blood flow
UBG	urobilinogen
UBI	ultraviolet blood irradiation
UBO	undetermined brain opacities (magnetic resonance imaging)

UC	ulcerative colitis unit clerk urea clearance (renal function test) urethral catheter usual care uterine contractions
U/C	urine culture
U & C	urethral and cervical usual and customary
U_{Ca}	urinary calcium
UCD	upper complete denture urine collection device usual childhood diseases
UCG	ultrasonic cardiogram urine chorionic gonadotropin
UCI	urethral catheter in usual childhood illnesses
UCN	undifferentiated carcinoma of the nasopharynx
UCO	urethral catheter out
UCPT	urinary coproporphyrin test
UCR	unconditioned reflex usual, customary, reasonable
UCS	unconditioned stimulus unconscious
UD	ulcerative dermatitis unipolar depression urethral discharge

UDE	undetermined etiology
UDO	undetermined origin
UDS	ultra-Doppler sonography
UE	upper extremity
UES	upper esophageal sphincter
UF	ultrafiltration
UFA	unesterified (free) fatty acids
UFC	urine free cortisol
UFO	unidentified foreign object
UFS	unilateral facial spasm
UG	urogenital
UGA	under general anesthesia
UGH	uveitis, glaucoma, hyphema
UGI	upper gastrointestinal (series)
UH	upper half
U24H	24-hour urine
UHF	ultrahigh frequency
UHV	ultrahigh voltage
U/I	unidentified
UIBC	unsaturated iron-binding capacity

UIQ	upper inner quadrant
UK	unknown urokinase
U_K	urinary potassium
UKM	urea kinetic modeling (dialysis)
UL	upper lobe
U & L	upper and lower
ULN	upper limits of normal
ULP	upper lid ptosis (ophthalmology)
ULQ	upper left quadrant
UM	upper motor (neuron) uterine monitor
U_{max}	maximum urinary osmolality
umb	umbilicus
UN	ulnar nerve urea nitrogen
U_{Na}	urinary sodium
uncomp	uncomplicated
uncond	unconditioned
uncor	uncorrected
ung	ointment (Latin: *unguentum*)
U_{NH4}	urinary ammonium

unilat	unilateral
unk	unknown
unoff	unofficial
UnS	unconditioned stimulus
unsat	unsatisfactory unsaturated
UO	urinary output
U/O	under observation
UONP	unilateral oculomotor nerve paralysis
UOQ	upper outer quadrant
$\mathbf{U_{osm}}$	urinary osmolality
UP	ureteropelvic uroporphyrin uteroplacental
U/P	urine-plasma ratio
$\mathbf{U_P}$	urinary phosphate
UPA	unpressurized aerosol (therapy) uteroplacental apoplexy
UPD	upper partial denture
UPEP	urine protein electrophoresis
UPI	uteroplacental insufficiency
UPJ	ureteropelvic junction

UPP	uteroplacental profilometry uvulopalatoplasty
UPPP	uvulopalatopharyngoplasty
UPS	ultraviolet photoelectron spectroscopy
UPT	urine pregnancy test uveoparotitis
UQ	upper quadrant (abdomen)
UR	unrelated upper respiratory utilization review
ur	urine
URC	upper respiratory condition
URD	upper respiratory disease
URF	uterine relaxing factor
URI	upper respiratory infection
URO	urology utilization review organization (hospital)
URQ	upper right quadrant (abdomen)
URS	ultrasonic renal scan urologic surgery
URT	upper respiratory tract
URTI	upper respiratory tract infection
URVD	unilateral renovascular disease

US	ultrasonic ultrasonography urine specimen
U/S	ultrasound
USA	unilateral spatial agnosia
USAS	uncomplicated supraclavicular aortic stenosis
USB	upper sternal border
USG	ultrasonograph
USI	urinary stress incontinence
USN	ultrasonic nebulizer
USO	unilateral salingo-oophorectomy
USP	United States Pharmacopeia
USR	unheated serum reagin (test)
USS	ultrasound scan
UT	untested untreated urinary tract
UTBG	unbound thyroxine-binding globulin
UTD	up-to-date
UTI	urinary tract infection
UTO	upper tibial osteotomy
UU	urine urobilinogen (laboratory/chemistry)

UUN	urine urea nitrogen
UV	ultraviolet umbilical vein urine volume
UVC	umbilical vein catheter
UVJ	ureterovesical junction
UVL	ultraviolet light
UVP	ultraviolet photometry
UVPP	uvulopalatopharyngoplasty
UVR	ultraviolet radiation
UZ	ultrasound

V

V	vaccinated valve vein vertex Vibrio (on bacteriology reports) virus vision voice volume volume of gas
$\dot{V}$	rate of gas flow volume of gas per unit of time
v	venous volt
V1, V2,...	chest lead 1, chest lead 2,... (electrocardiograph)
VA	vacuum aspiration ventricular aneurysm ventriculoatrial (shunt) vertebral artery Veterans Affairs (hospital) visual acuity (eye examination)
V_A	volume of alveolar gas
$\dot{V}_A$	alveolar ventilation
V_a	volume of arterial gas
VAC	vincristine, actinomycin (D), cyclophosphamide (chemotherapy)
vac	vacuum

vacc	vaccinate
VACTERL	vertebral, anal, cardiac, tracheo-esophageal, renal, limb (syndrome)
VAD	ventricular assistive device vincristine, adriamycin, dexamethasone (chemotherapy)
VAE	venous air embolism
VAg	visual agnosia
vag hyst	vaginal hysterectomy
VAH	Veterans Affairs Hospital virilizing adrenal hyperplasia
VAHS	virus-associated hemophagocytic syndrome
VAK	vestibuloauditory keratitis
VAMC	Veterans Affairs Medical Center
VAMP	vincristine, amethopterin, 6-mercapto-purine and prednisone
VAP	variant angina pectoris ventilator-associated pneumonia
V_A/Qc	ratio of alveolar ventilation to pulmonary capillary perfusion
var	variable various
VAS	ventriculoatrial shunt
VASC	Verbal Auditory Screen for Children

vasc vascular

VAT ventricular activation time
ventricular pacing, atrial sensing, triggered mode (pacemaker)
virilizing adrenal tumor
visual apperception test

VATS video-assisted thoracoscopic surgery

VB vaginal bleeding
vertebrobasilar (arteries)
viable birth
vinblastine

VBAC vaginal birth after cesarean (section)

VBAO vertebrobasilar artery occlusion

VBC vincristine, bleomycin, cisplatin (chemotherapy)

VBG venoaortocoronary artery bypass graft
vertical banded gastroplasty

VBI vertebrobasilar insufficiency

VBL vinblastine

VBM vinblastine, bleomycin, methotrexate (chemotherapy)

VBS vertebrobasilar system (stroke)

VC color vision (eye examination)
vaginal candidiasis
vascular catheterization
vasoconstriction
vena cava
venous capacitance

VC *(cont)*	ventilatory capacity visual cortex vital capacity vocal cord
V/C	ventilation-circulation ratio
V_c	pulmonary capillary gas volume
VCA	viral capsid antigen
V_{CF}	mean fiber-shortening rate
VCG	vectorcardiogram
VCO_2	carbon dioxide output
VCP	vincristine, cyclophosphamide, prednisone (chemotherapy)
VCR	vincristine sulfate
VCS	ventricular conduction system
VCT	venous clotting time
VCU	voiding cystourethrogram (procedure, urology)
VD	vasodilator venereal disease
V_D	volume of dead space gas
V & D	vertigo and deafness
VDA	venous digital angiogram vertigo, diplopia, ataxia visual discriminatory acuity

VDC	vasodilator center
VDEL	Venereal Disease Experimental Laboratory
VDF	ventricular diastolic fragmentation
VDG	venereal disease, gonorrhea
VDH	valvular disease of the heart
VDM	vasodepressor material
VDP	vincristine, daunorubicin, prednisone (chemotherapy)
$\mathbf{V_D rb}$	rebreathing ventilation
VDRL	Venereal Disease Research Laboratory
VDS	vasodilator substance venereal disease, syphilis
$\mathbf{V_D/V_T}$	ratio of dead space ventilation to total ventilation
VE	vaginal examination ventilatory effort viral encephalitis visual examination
$\mathbf{V_E}$	volume of expired gas
$\mathbf{\dot{V}_E}$	minute volume
V & E	vinethene and ether (anesthetic agents)
VEA	ventricular ectopic arrhythmia
VEB	ventricular ectopic beat

vect	vector
VEF	ventricular ejection fraction
VEM	vasoexcitor material
vent	ventilation ventral ventricle
ventric	ventricular
VEP	visual evoked potentials voluntary eye propulsion
VER	ventricular escape rhythm visual evoked response (neurological test)
vert	vertebra vertical
ves	vessel
vesic	vesicular
vest	vestibular
VF	ventricular fibrillation visual field (eye examination) vocal fremitus
VFC	ventricular function curve
VFD	visual field defect
VFib	ventricular fibrillation
VFP	ventricular fluid pressure vitreous fluorophotometry

VG	vein graft ventricular gallop (rhythm)
V/G	very good
VGM	ventriculogram
VH	vaginal hysterectomy ventricular hypertrophy viral hepatitis vitreous hemorrhage
VHD	valvular heart disease
VHDL	very high density lipoprotein
VHF	very high frequency visual half-field (eye examination)
VHL	von Hippel-Lindau (disease)
VI	visual impairment volume index
V_I	volume of inspired gas
VIA	virus-inactivating agent
Vib	Vibrio (on laboratory reports)
vib	vibration
VIC	vasoinhibitory center
VID	videodensitometry
VIG	vaccinia immune globulin
VIM	video intensification microscopy

VIP	vasoactive intestinal peptide venous impedance plethysmography very important person voluntary interruption of pregnancy
VIR	virology
VIS	vaginal irrigation smear
vis	vision visitor
VISC	vitreous infusion suction cutter
visc	visceral viscous
VIT	venom immunotherapy
Vit	vitamin
vit	vital
VJ	ventriculojugular (shunt)
VL	vision, left (eye)
$\mathbf{V_L}$	lung volume
VLBW	very low birth weight
VLCD	very low calorie diet
VLDL	very low density lipoproteins
VLM	visceral larva migrans
VLP	ventriculolumbar perfusion
VLS	vanishing lung syndrome

VM	Venturi mask vestibular membrane viral myocarditis
VMA	vanillylmandelic acid (assay)
V_{max}	maximum velocity
VMCG	vector magnetocardiogram
VMHL	ventromedial hypothalamic lesions
VMN	ventromedial nuclei
VMT	visceral malignant tumor
VN	visiting nurse
V/O	verbal order
VO_2	oxygen consumption
VOD	vision, right eye (eye examination)
vol	volume voluntary
VO_2 max	maximum oxygen consumption
VOO	ventricular pacing, no sensing, no other function (pacemaker)
VOS	vision, left eye (eye examination)
VOU	vision, each eye (eye examination)
VP	vasopressin venipuncture venous pressure ventriculoperitoneal (shunt)

V_P	plasma volume
vp	vapor pressure
V & P	vagotomy and pyloroplasty ventilation and perfusion
VPA	valproic acid
VPB	ventricular premature beat
VPC	ventricular premature contraction
VPD	ventricular premature depolarization
VPI	velopharyngeal insufficiency
VPLS	ventilation-perfusion lung scan
VPRC	volume of packed red cells
VPS	vascular pulmonic stenosis
vps	vibrations per second
V/Q	ventilation-perfusion ratio
VR	valve replacement vascular resistance venous return ventral root ventricular rate vision, right (eye) vocal resonance vocational rehabilitation
VRI	viral respiratory infection
VRP	very reliable product (hospital)

VRT volume replacement therapy

VRV ventricular residual volume

VS vagal stimulation
vascular spasm
vascular surgery
venesection
vesicular sounds
vesicular stomatitis

V/S vital signs

vs versus
vibration-second

VSD ventricular septal defect (heart)

VSM vascular smooth muscle

VSR venous stasis retinopathy

VSS vital signs stable

VSW ventricular stroke work

VT venous thrombosis
ventricular tachycardia
video telemetry

V_T tidal volume (pulmonary function test)
total ventilation

V_t volume of pulmonary parenchymal tissue

V & T volume and tension (pulse)

V_TA alveolar tidal volume

VTE venous thromboembolism

V_{TG}	volume of thoracic gas
VTI	volume thickness index
V_TM	mechanical tidal volume
VTP	voluntary termination of pregnancy
vtx	vertex
VU	vesicouterogram
VUR	vesicoureteral reflux
VV	varicose veins
vv	veins
v/v	volume for volume
V & V	vulva and vagina
VVF	vesicovaginal fistula
VVI	ventricular pacing, ventricular sensing, inhibited mode
VVT	ventricular pacing, ventricular sensing, triggered mode
VWD	von Willebrand's disease
VWF	von Willebrand factor
vx	vertex
VZ	varicella-zoster
VZIG	varicella-zoster immune globulin

VZV varicella-zoster virus

W

W	water weight white widow (widower) width wife
W+	weakly positive (laboratory)
w	week with
WA	while awake
WAB	Western Aphasia Battery (test)
WAIS-R	Wechsler Adult Intelligence Scale — Revised (psychological test)
WAP	wandering atrial pacemaker
WAR	whole abdominal radiation
Wass	Wassermann (syphilis test)
WB	water baby (nephrogenic diabetes insipidus) water bottle weight-bearing western blot (blood test for AIDS) whole blood whole body
Wb	weber (unit of magnetic flux)
WBAPT	whole blood activated partial thromboplastin (time)

WBAT	weight-bearing as tolerated
WBC	white blood (cell) count
WBC/hpf	white blood cells per high power field (on urinalysis reports)
WBCT	whole blood clotting time
WBH	whole body hematocrit
WBPT	whole blood partial thromboplastin (time)
WBR	whole body radiation
WBS	whole body scan
WBT	western blot test (AIDS blood test) wet bulb temperature
WC	ward clerk wheelchair white count whooping cough
WC/B	will call back
WCCD	white cell count with differential
WCE	work capacity evaluation
WD	well-developed well-differentiated wet dressing
Wd	ward
wd	wound
w/d	warm and dry

WDA	wrist disarticulation
WDHA	watery diarrhea with hypokalemia and achlorhydria
wds	wounds
WD/WN	well-developed, well-nourished
WE	wandering edema
w/e	weekend
WEE	western equine encephalitis
WF	Weil-Felix (reaction) white female
WFEx	Williams flexion exercises
WFL	within functional limits
WGM	Wegener's granulomatosis
wgt	weight
WH	well-healed well-hydrated
WHR	waist-to-hip ratio
WHVP	wedged hepatic venous pressure
WIC	Women, Infants and Children (program)
wid	widow (widower)
WISC-R	Wechsler Intelligence Scale for Children—Revised

WK	Wernicke-Korsakoff (syndrome)
wk	weak
WL	waiting list
wl	wavelength
WLD	work-loss day
WLT	waterload test (procedure/endocrinology)
WM	wet mount (bacteriology) white male whole milk
WMP	weight management program
WMS	Wechsler Memory Scale
WMX	whirlpool, massage, exercise (physical therapy)
WN	well-nourished
WNF	well-nourished female
WNL	within normal limits
WNM	well-nourished male
W/O	water in oil written order
w/o	weeks old without
WOL	weakness of limbs
WP	wrong position (radiology)

w/p whirlpool (physical therapy)

WPM wandering pacemaker

WPP wide pulse pressure

WPW Wolff-Parkinson-White (syndrome)

WR Wassermann reaction
water retention
weakly reactive

wr wrist

WRVP wedged renal vein pressure

w/s water-soluble
watt-seconds

WSU weak-stream urination

WT water temperature
Wilm's tumor

wt weight
wisdom teeth

w/u work-up

WUP Waldenstroem's uveoparotitis

WV whispered voice

w/v weight per volume

WV-MBC ratio of walking ventilation to maximum breathing capacity

WWAC walks with aid of cane

X

X	cross (transverse) crossmatch magnification removal start of anesthesia times unknown
$\bar{X}$	except
Ⓧ	end of anesthesia
x	axis (of cylindrical lens)
$\bar{x}$	mean
x3, x4,...	three times, four times,...
Xa	chiasma
Xaa	unknown amino acid
Xan	xanthomatosis
XAT	xylose absorption test
XBT	xylose breath test
XC	excretory cystogram
XCCE	extracapsular cataract extraction
XD	X-linked dominant
x2d, x3d,...	for two days, for three days,... (medication orders)
XEF	excess ejection fraction

XES	x-ray energy spectrometry
XGP	xanthogranulomatous pyelonephritis
XH	extra high
XLH	x-linked hydrocephalus
XLP	x-linked lymphoproliferative (disorder)
XM	crossmatch (laboratory/blood bank)
XMM	xeromammography
XN	night blindness
XOM	extraocular movement
XP	xeroderma pigmentosum
XPS	xiphoid process syndrome x-ray photoemission spectroscopy
XR	x-linked recessive
XRD	x-ray diffraction
XRT	x-ray therapy
XS	corneal scar cross section
XSA	cross-sectional area xenograph surface area
XSLR	crossed straight leg raising
XT	exercise test exotropia (eye examination)

XU excretory urogram

XUV ultra-ultraviolet

XX double strength
normal female chromosome type

XY normal male chromosome type

Xyl xylose

Xylo xylocaine

Y

Y	year young
YACP	young adult chronic patient
YAG	yttrium-aluminum-garnet (laser)
YE	yeast extract yellow enzyme
YEH_2	reduced yellow enzyme
yel	yellow
Yer	Yersinia (on bacteriology reports)
YET	youth effectiveness training (psychiatry)
YF	yellow fever
Y-F	Y-fracture
YJV	yellow jacket venom
YLC	youngest living child
YLS	years of life saved
YMA	yellow mutant albinism
YNS	yellow nail syndrome
y/o	years old
YOB	year of birth
YOD	year of death

YORA	younger-onset rheumatoid arthritis
YP	yeast phase yield pressure
Y-P	Y-plasty
YPLL	years of potential life lost
YR	Young's rule (dosage)
yr	year
YS	yellow spot (retina) yolk sac Yoshida's sarcoma
Y-S	Y-set (surgery)
YSC	yolk sac carcinoma
YSP	Yergason's sign positive (test for tendonitis)
YTD	year to date
YV	yellow vernix (obstetrics)

Z

Z	impedance zero zone
Z, Z', Z"	increasing degrees of contraction
ZAT	Zondek-Aschheim test (gynecology)
ZCE	Zinsser-Cole-Engman syndrome (dermatology)
ZD	zero discharge
Z/D	zero defects
ZDS	Zung Depression Scale (psychiatry)
ZEEP	zero end-expiratory pressure
ZES	Zollinger-Ellison syndrome
ZESR	zeta erythrocyte sedimentation rate
ZF	zona fasciculata (adrenal cortex)
ZFT	zinc flocculation test
ZG	zona glomerulosa (adrenal cortex)
ZIFT	zygote intrafallopian transfer (fertilization technique)
ZIG	zoster immune globulin
ZIP	zoster immune plasma
ZMC	zygomaticomaxillary complex

ZNS	Ziehl-Neelsen stain
ZnSR	zinc sedimentation rate
Z-P	Z-plasty
ZR	zona reticularis (adrenal cortex)
ZSB	zero stool since birth
ZSR	zeta sedimentation rate
ZTT	zinc turbidity test
ZTX	zootoxin
ZV	zidovudine (AIDS treatment drug)

SYMBOLS

+ or ⊕	acid reaction add, added to and convex lens excess increased markedly impaired pulse mildly positive mildly severe plus positive present slight trace or reaction (laboratory tests) sluggish reflexes (neurology/orthopedics) uncertain or uncommon mode of inheritance (genetics)
(+)	significant
(+)ive	positive
++	average reflexes (neurology/orthopedics) moderately impaired pulse moderate pain moderately positive or severe noticeable trace or reaction (laboratory tests)
+++	increased reflexes (neurology/orthopedics) moderate amount moderately hyperactive reflexes (neurology/orthopedics) moderate reaction (laboratory tests) moderately severe pain slightly impaired pulse
++++	large amount (laboratory tests) markedly severe pain

++++ *(cont)*	normal pulse pronounced reaction (laboratory tests) very brisk reflexes (neurology/orthopedics)
++/+	2 plus on the right, 1 plus on the left
±	doubtful either positive or negative indefinite possibly significant questionable suggestive very slight trace (or reaction) with or without
± to +	minimal pain
(±)	possibly significant
$\dot{+}$	direct sum
– or ⊖	absent alkaline reaction concave lens decreased deficiency minus negative none subtract without
(–)	insignificant
+ rct	acid reaction
– rct	alkaline reaction
=	equal to

Symbols

$\simeq$	similar or equal
$\approx$	approximately or nearly equal
$\sim$	approximate proportionate to similar
$\nsim$	not similar
$\not\simeq$	not similar or equal
$\not\approx$	not approximately equal
$\equiv$	identical
$\propto$	proportional
$>$	from which is derived greater than
$<$	less than
$\geq$	greater than or equal to
$\leq$	less than or equal to
$\ngeq$	neither greater than nor equal to
$\ngtr$	not greater than
$\nless$	not less than
$\nprec$	does not precede
$\npreceq$	neither precedes nor equals
∞	infinity
$::$	as

∷ *(cont)*	breakage and reunion (genetics/laboratory) proportionate to
∵	because
∴	therefore
∠	angle flexion flexor
∪	logical sum union
⊂	is contained in
△	anion gap change heat increment prism diopter
↑	above alive elevated enlarged gas greater than high improved increase rising superior position up upper
↓	below dead decreased deficiency or deficit

↓ *(cont)*	depressed deteriorated or deteriorating diminished down falling inferior position less than low, lower or lowered normal plantar reflexes precipitate restricted
→	approaches limit of demonstrates direction of flow or reaction distal followed by indicates is due to no change produces progressing radiates to results in reveals shows or showed to to the right toward transfer to vector yields
←	caused by derived from direction of flow or reaction is due to produced by proximal resulting from

Symbols

↔	stable to and from unchanging widened width
↑↑	extensor response, Babinski sign (neurological examination) testes undescended
↓↓	both down down bilaterally plantar response, Babinski sign (neurological examination) testes descended
↑↓	reversible reaction up and down
↑c	increase due to chemical interference during assay
↓c	decrease due to chemical interference during assay
↑g	increasing rising
↓g	decreasing falling
↑ICP	increased intracranial pressure
↑v	increase due to in vivo effect (laboratory)
↓v	decrease due to in vivo effect (laboratory)
↗	deviated displaced increasing

Symbols

↙	decreased
↖	direction
∨	below deficiency depressed deteriorating inferior less than or systolic blood pressure (on anesthesiology records)
∧	above and diastolic blood pressure (on anesthesiology records) elevated enlarged greater than improved superior upper
○	respirations (on anesthesiology records) living female normal female right ear-masked air conduction threshold
●	affected female deceased female pulse rate (on anesthesiology records)
○○	male
⊙⊙	biennial
⊗	end of anesthesia end of operation (on anesthesia records)

Symbols

∅	death, female empty set none
⊖	normal
⊙	annual carrier of sex-linked recessive gold start of operation (on anesthesia records) sun
⦽	abortion or stillbirth with sex unspecified
■	affected male deceased male
□	brother father left ear-masked air conduction threshold living male normal male son
(□)	adopted
⧄	death, male
◇	sex unknown sex unspecified
♀	copper female female sex Venus
♂	iron male male sex Mars

Symbols

√	flexion observe for urine voided
√c̄	check with
√d	checked observed
√qs	voided quantity sufficient
℞	prescription take
†	dead death deceased died moderate severity normally active reflexes (neurology/orthopedics)
?	doubtful equivocal reflexes (neurology/orthopedics) flicker reflexes (neurology/orthopedics) possible questionable question of suggested severity unknown
*	birth multiplication sign in genetics not verified presumed supposed
′	foot minute

′ (cont)	prime univalent
″	bivalent ditto inch second
@	at
#	fracture gauge has been done or given number pound(s) weight
[	right ear-masked bone conduction threshold
]	left ear-masked bone conduction threshold
/	divided by either meaning extension fraction of organic per to
:	is to ratio
(	concave
)	convex
°	degree severity of burns or wounds

° *(cont)*	temperature time (hour)
0	completely absent pulse no muscular contraction no reflex response (neurology/orthopedics)
1	trace of muscle contraction
1+	low normal reflexes (neurology/orthopedics) markedly impaired pulse
1°	first degree one hour primary
2	active movement of body part with gravity eliminated (neurology/orthopedics)
2+	average reflexes (neurology/orthopedics) moderately impaired pulse
2°	because of due to second degree two hours
3	active movement of body part against gravity (neurology/orthopedics)
3+	brisk reflexes (neurology/orthopedics) slightly impaired pulse
3°	tertiary third degree three hours
4	active movement against gravity and some resistance (neurology/orthopedics)

Symbols

4+	normal pulse very brisk reflexes (neurology/orthopedics)
4/6	loud heart murmur
5/6	very loud heart murmur
6/6	extremely loud heart murmur
24°	24 hours
$\dot{\top}$	one
$\ddot{\top}$	two
$\dddot{\top}$	three
1X	once
2X	twice
2ndry	secondary
ʒ	dram (teaspoonful, approx 5 ml)
*f*ʒ	fluid dram (tablespoon, approx 15 ml)
℥	ounce
½℥	half-ounce
f℥	fluid ounce
α	alpha particle angular acceleration heavy chain of immunoglobulin A is proportional to optical rotation (chemistry) prefix denoting first in a series

α *(cont)*	probability of type I error (statistics) significance level solubility coefficient (Bunson's)
αCD	alpha-chain disease
α-GLUC	alpha-glucosidase
α-LP	alpha-lipoprotein
β	beta particle buffer capacity prefix denoting second in a series probability of type II error (statistics)
β2m	beta_2 microglobulin
γ	done gamma chain of fetal hemoglobin heavy chain of immunoglobulin G photon (gamma ray) plasma protein (globulin) prefix denoting third in a series
γG	immunoglobulin G
γGT	gamma-aminobutyric acid
γ-HCD	gamma heavy chain disease
△	absense of heat in a reaction centrad prism change delta gap diagnosis head increment prism diopter right ear-masked air conduction threshold sulfur

Symbols

△*A*	change in absorbance
△dB	change in decibels (otorhinolaryngology)
△EF	ejection fraction response
△P	change in pressure (ophthalmology)
△pH	change in pH
△ scan	delta scan (computed tomography scan)
△t	time interval
△9 THC	delta-9-tetrahydrocannabinol
δ	delta chain of hemoglobin heavy chain of immunoglobulin D prefix denoting fourth in a series
ϵ	dielectric constant heavy chain of immunoglobulin E molar absorptivity molar extinction coefficient prefix denoting fifth in a series specific absorptivity
η	absolute viscosity apparent or dynamic velocity
Θ	kinetic constant thermodynamic temperature
θ	angular coordinate variable customary temperature latent trait (statistics) temperature interval
κ	magnetic susceptibility

λ	craniometric point decay constant homosexuality junction of lambdoid and sagittal sutures (craniotomy) thermal conductivity wavelength
μ	chemical potential dynamic viscosity electrophoretic mobility heavy chain of immunoglobulin M magnetic moment mass absorption coefficient micro- (10^{-6}) micrometer (or micron) (one thousandth of a millimeter) mutation rate statistical mean
μA	microampere (one thousandth of an ampere)
μb	microbar (also μbar)
μC	microcoulomb (also μcoul)
μc	microcurie (also μCi)
μch	microcurie-hour (also μCi-hr)
μEq	microequivalent
μF (and μf)	microfarad
μγ	microgamma (also called micromicrogram and picogram)
μg	microgram (one-millionth of a gram)

Symbols

μGy	microgray
μH	microhenry
μHg	micrometer of mercury (also μmHg)
μin	microinch
μIU	one-millionth International Unit
μL (and μl)	microliter (one-millionth of a liter)
μM	micromolar
μm	micrometer micromilli-
μmm	micromillimeter (also called nanometer)
μmμ	meson
mμ	millimicro-
mμc	millimicrocurie (also called nanocurie)
mμg	millimicrogram (also called nanogram)
μmol/L	micromoles per liter
μN	micronormal
μOsm	micro-osmole
μ/p	mass attenuation coefficient
μR (and μr)	microroentgen
μs (and μsec)	microsecond
μU	microunit

μV	microvolt
μW (and μw)	microwatt
μμ	micromicro- micromicron (10^{-12})
μμc (and μμCi)	micromicrocurie (also called picocurie)
μμF	micromicrofarad
μμg	micromicrogram (also called picogram)
ν	frequency kinematic viscosity
π	3.1416 (ratio of circumference of a circle to its diameter) osmotic pressure
ρ	correlation coefficient electric charge density mass density population correlation coefficient
Σ	foaminess sigmoid sum of syphilis
σ	conductivity difference one-thousandth of a second (millisecond) reflection coefficient standard deviation stress surface tension wave number
$σ^2$	variance for a normal distribution

Symbols

σD	standard deviation of difference
τ	life (of pharmaceuticals and radioactive isotopes) mean life relaxation time shear stress spectral transmittance torque transmission coefficient
τ½	half-life (of pharmaceuticals and radioactive isotopes)
ø	magnetic flux osmotic coefficient
χ^2	chi-square (test of statistical significance)
χe	susceptibility (electricity)
χm	magnetic susceptibility
Ψ	psychiatric
ψ	pseudo wave function
ω	angular frequency angular velocity

New Abbreviations

New Abbreviations

New Abbreviations

New Abbreviations

New Abbreviations

New Abbreviations